# Health Literacy and Numeracy

## WORKSHOP SUMMARY

Melissa G. French, *Rapporteur*

Roundtable on Health Literacy

Board on Population Health and Public Health Practice

### INSTITUTE OF MEDICINE
*OF THE NATIONAL ACADEMIES*

THE NATIONAL ACADEMIES PRESS
Washington, D.C.
**www.nap.edu**

THE NATIONAL ACADEMIES PRESS    500 Fifth Street, NW    Washington, DC 20001

NOTICE: The workshop that is the subject of this workshop summary was approved by the Governing Board of the National Research Council, whose members are drawn from the councils of the National Academy of Sciences, the National Academy of Engineering, and the Institute of Medicine.

This activity was supported by contracts between the National Academy of Sciences and the Agency for Healthcare Research and Quality (HHSP233200900537P); the American College of Physicians Foundation; America's Health Insurance Plans; the California Dental Association; the East Bay Community Foundation (Kaiser Permanente); Eli Lilly and Company; the Health Resources and Services Administration (HHSH25034004T); Humana; Johnson & Johnson; Merck and Co., Inc.; the North Shore–Long Island Jewish Health System; the Office of Disease Prevention and Health Promotion; and the UnitedHealth Group. The views presented in this publication are those of the rapporteur and do not necessarily reflect the views of the organizations or agencies that provided support for the activity.

International Standard Book Number-13:  978-0-309-29980-0
International Standard Book Number-10:  0-309-29980-2

Additional copies of this workshop summary are available for sale from the National Academies Press, 500 Fifth Street, NW, Keck 360, Washington, DC 20001; (800) 624-6242 or (202) 334-3313; http://www.nap.edu.

For more information about the Institute of Medicine, visit the IOM home page at: www.iom.edu.

The serpent has been a symbol of long life, healing, and knowledge among almost all cultures and religions since the beginning of recorded history. The serpent adopted as a logotype by the Institute of Medicine is a relief carving from ancient Greece, now held by the Staatliche Museen in Berlin.

Suggested citation: IOM (Institute of Medicine). 2014. *Health Literacy and Numeracy: Workshop Summary*. Washington, DC: The National Academies Press.

*"Knowing is not enough; we must apply.*
*Willing is not enough; we must do."*
—Goethe

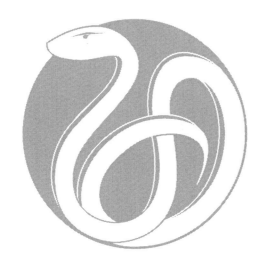

# INSTITUTE OF MEDICINE
## *OF THE NATIONAL ACADEMIES*

**Advising the Nation. Improving Health.**

# THE NATIONAL ACADEMIES
*Advisers to the Nation on Science, Engineering, and Medicine*

The **National Academy of Sciences** is a private, nonprofit, self-perpetuating society of distinguished scholars engaged in scientific and engineering research, dedicated to the furtherance of science and technology and to their use for the general welfare. Upon the authority of the charter granted to it by the Congress in 1863, the Academy has a mandate that requires it to advise the federal government on scientific and technical matters. Dr. Ralph J. Cicerone is president of the National Academy of Sciences.

The **National Academy of Engineering** was established in 1964, under the charter of the National Academy of Sciences, as a parallel organization of outstanding engineers. It is autonomous in its administration and in the selection of its members, sharing with the National Academy of Sciences the responsibility for advising the federal government. The National Academy of Engineering also sponsors engineering programs aimed at meeting national needs, encourages education and research, and recognizes the superior achievements of engineers. Dr. C. D. Mote, Jr., is president of the National Academy of Engineering.

The **Institute of Medicine** was established in 1970 by the National Academy of Sciences to secure the services of eminent members of appropriate professions in the examination of policy matters pertaining to the health of the public. The Institute acts under the responsibility given to the National Academy of Sciences by its congressional charter to be an adviser to the federal government and, upon its own initiative, to identify issues of medical care, research, and education. Dr. Harvey V. Fineberg is president of the Institute of Medicine.

The **National Research Council** was organized by the National Academy of Sciences in 1916 to associate the broad community of science and technology with the Academy's purposes of furthering knowledge and advising the federal government. Functioning in accordance with general policies determined by the Academy, the Council has become the principal operating agency of both the National Academy of Sciences and the National Academy of Engineering in providing services to the government, the public, and the scientific and engineering communities. The Council is administered jointly by both Academies and the Institute of Medicine. Dr. Ralph J. Cicerone and Dr. C. D. Mote, Jr., are chair and vice chair, respectively, of the National Research Council.

**www.national-academies.org**

# PLANNING COMMITTEE ON HEALTH LITERACY AND NUMERACY[1]

**ANDREA APTER,** Professor of Medicine, University of Pennsylvania

**SUSAN PISANO,** Vice President of Communications, America's Health Insurance Plans

**LYNN QUINCY,** Senior Policy Analyst, Consumers Union

**RIMA RUDD,** Department of Society, Human Development and Health, Harvard School of Public Health

**STEVEN RUSH,** Director, Health Literacy Innovations Program, UnitedHealth Group

**WINSTON F. WONG,** Medical Director, Community Benefit, Disparities Improvement and Quality Initiatives, Kaiser Permanente

---

[1] Institute of Medicine planning committees are solely responsible for organizing the workshop, identifying topics, and choosing speakers. The responsibility for the published workshop summary rests with the workshop rapporteur and the institution.

# ROUNDTABLE ON HEALTH LITERACY[1]

**GEORGE ISHAM** (*Chair*), Medical Director and Chief Health Officer, HealthPartners
**WILMA ALVARADO-LITTLE,** Director, Community Engagement/Outreach Center for the Elimination of Minority Health Disparities, University of Albany
**CINDY BRACH,** Senior Health Policy Researcher, Center for Delivery, Organization, and Markets, Agency for Healthcare Research and Quality
**GEMIRALD DAUS,** Public Health Analyst, Health Resources and Services Administration Office of Health Equity, U.S. Department of Health and Human Services
**DARREN DEWALT,** Associate Professor of Medicine, University of North Carolina at Chapel Hill
**BENARD P. DREYER,** Professor of Pediatrics, New York University School of Medicine, and Chair, American Academy of Pediatrics Health Literacy Program Advisory Committee
**ELIZABETH FOWLER,** Vice President, Global Health Policy, Johnson & Johnson
**LAURIE FRANCIS,** Senior Director of Clinic Operations and Quality, Oregon Primary Care Association
**LORI HALL,** Consultant, Health Education, Eli Lilly and Company
**LINDA HARRIS,** Team Leader, Health Communication and eHealth Team, Office of Disease Prevention and Health Promotion, U.S. Department of Health and Human Services
**BETSY L. HUMPHREYS,** Deputy Director, National Library of Medicine, National Institutes of Health
**MARGARET LOVELAND,** Global Medical Affairs, Merck & Co., Inc.
**PATRICK McGARRY,** Assistant Division Director, Scientific Activities Division, American Academy of Family Physicians
**RUTH PARKER,** Professor of Medicine, Emory University School of Medicine
**TERRI ANN PARNELL,** Vice President, Health Literacy and Patient Education, North Shore–Long Island Jewish Health System
**KIM PARSON,** Consumer Experience, Humana, Inc.
**KAVITA PATEL,** Managing Director for Clinical Transformation and Delivery, The Brookings Institution

---

[1] Institute of Medicine forums and roundtables do not issue, review, or approve individual documents. The responsibility for the published workshop summary rests with the workshop rapporteur and the institution.

CLARENCE PEARSON, Consultant, Global Health Leadership and Management
SUSAN PISANO, Vice President of Communications, America's Health Insurance Plans
ANDREW PLEASANT, Health Literacy and Research Director, Canyon Ranch Institute
LINDSEY ROBINSON, President, California Dental Association
RIMA RUDD, Department of Society, Human Development and Health, Harvard School of Public Health
STEVEN RUSH, Director, Health Literacy Innovations Program, UnitedHealth Group
PAUL M. SCHYVE, Senior Vice President, The Joint Commission
PATRICK WAYTE, Vice President, Marketing and Health Education, American Heart Association
WINSTON F. WONG, Medical Director, Community Benefit, Disparities Improvement and Quality Initiatives, Kaiser Permanente

*IOM Staff*

LYLA M. HERNANDEZ, Roundtable Director
MELISSA G. FRENCH, Associate Program Officer
ANDREW LEMERISE, Research Associate
ANGELA MARTIN, Senior Program Assistant
ROSE MARIE MARTINEZ, Director, Board on Population Health and Public Health Practice

# Reviewers

This workshop summary has been reviewed in draft form by individuals chosen for their diverse perspectives and technical expertise, in accordance with procedures approved by the National Research Council's Report Review Committee. The purpose of this independent review is to provide candid and critical comments that will assist the institution in making its published workshop summary as sound as possible and to ensure that the workshop summary meets institutional standards for objectivity, evidence, and responsiveness to the study charge. The review comments and draft manuscript remain confidential to protect the integrity of the process. We wish to thank the following individuals for their review of this workshop summary:

**CRYSTAL DURAN,** Clinical Program Manager, Customer Experience, Cigna

**ELIZABETH HAHN,** Associate Professor, Department of Medical Social Sciences, Northwestern University

**AILEEN KANTOR,** Vice President, Marketing, Health Literacy Innovations

**SUSAN PISANO,** Vice President of Communications, America's Health Insurance Plans

Although the reviewers listed above have provided many constructive comments and suggestions, they did not see the final draft of the workshop summary before its release. The review of this workshop summary was overseen by **Georges Benjamin,** American Public Health Association. Appointed by the National Research Council, he was responsible for making certain that an independent examination of this workshop summary was carried out in accordance with institutional procedures and that all review comments were carefully considered. Responsibility for the final content of this workshop summary rests entirely with the rapporteur and the institution.

# Acknowledgments

The sponsors of the Institute of Medicine Roundtable on Health Literacy made it possible to plan and conduct the workshop, Health Literacy and Numeracy. Sponsors from the U.S. Department of Health and Human Services are the Agency for Healthcare Research and Quality; the Health Resources and Services Administration; and the Office of Disease Prevention and Health Promotion. Non-federal sponsorship was provided by the American College of Physicians Foundation; America's Health Insurance Plans; the California Dental Association; the East Bay Community Foundation (Kaiser Permanente); Eli Lilly and Company; Humana; Johnson & Johnson; Merck and Co., Inc.; the North Shore–Long Island Jewish Health System; and the UnitedHealth Group.

The roundtable wishes to express its gratitude to the following speakers for their interesting and thoughtful presentations: Jessica Ancker, Andrea Apter, Terry Davis, Lynda Ginsburg, Marguerite Holloway, Robert Krughoff, Ellen Peters, Lynn Quincy, Michael Wolf, and Brian Zikmund-Fisher. The roundtable also wishes to extend its appreciation to the planning committee members: Andrea Apter, Susan Pisano, Lynn Quincy, Rima Rudd, Steven Rush, and Winston Wong.

# Contents

APPENDIXES

# Boxes, Figures, and Tables

# 1

# Introduction[1]

The Board on Population Health and Public Health Practice of the Institute of Medicine established the Roundtable on Health Literacy to foster dialogue and discussion to advance the field of health literacy and to improve the translation of research findings to health care, education, and policy. The roundtable strives to enhance mutual understanding of health literacy among the health community and the general public, and to provide a mechanism that fosters collaboration among stakeholders. To accomplish its purpose, the roundtable brings together leaders from academia, industry, government, foundations, and associations as well as representatives of patients and consumers who have an interest and role in improving health literacy. It also commissions papers and conducts workshops to inform its meetings.

Although health literacy is commonly defined as an individual trait, it does not depend on the skills of individuals alone. Health literacy is the product of the interaction between individuals' capacities *and* the health literacy-related demands and complexities of the health care system. Specifically, the ability to understand, evaluate, and use numbers is important to making informed health care choices.

---

[1] The planning committee's role was limited to planning the workshop, and the workshop summary has been prepared by the workshop rapporteur as a factual summary of what occurred at the workshop. Statements, recommendations, and opinions expressed are those of individual presenters and participants, and are not necessarily endorsed or verified by the Institute of Medicine, and they should not be construed as reflecting any group consensus.

The Roundtable on Health Literacy commissioned a paper on numeracy skills that addressed the following questions:

1.  What does research show about people's numeracy skill levels?
2.  What kinds of numeracy skills are needed to select a health plan, choose treatments, and understand medication instructions?
3.  What do we know about how providers should communicate with those with low numeracy skills?

On July 18, 2013, the roundtable conducted a workshop that featured the presentation of the commissioned paper by its authors (see Appendix A for the commissioned paper). Other presenters were invited to speak on a number of topics related to numeracy, including the effects of ill health on cognitive capacity, issues with communication of health information to the public, and communicating numeric information for decision making. The workshop was organized into four panels of speakers, each followed by a brief discussion. The following chapters of the workshop summary are organized by panel presentations. The moderator of the workshop was roundtable member Paul Schyve.

The workshop (see Appendix B for the agenda) was organized by an independent planning committee in accordance with the procedures of the National Academy of Sciences. The planning committee members were Andrea Apter, Susan Pisano, Lynn Quincy, Rima Rudd, Steve Rush, and Winston Wong. The role of the workshop planning committee was limited to planning the workshop. Unlike a consensus report, a workshop summary may not contain conclusions and recommendations, except as expressed by and attributed to individual presenters and participants. Therefore, this summary has been prepared by the workshop rapporteur as a factual summary of what occurred at the workshop.

# 2

# Overview of Numeracy

The first panel was separated into two sections, each followed by a brief discussion section. It began with a presentation defining the concept of numeracy by Lynda Ginsburg, an educational researcher at Rutgers University. This was followed by the presentation of the commissioned paper by Ellen Peters, a professor in the Department of Psychology at Ohio State University. The last speaker was Terry Davis, a professor of medicine and pediatrics at Louisiana State University Health Sciences Center in Shreveport. Davis spoke about her personal experience with numeracy and health literacy as a patient.

## WHAT IS NUMERACY?: IT'S MORE THAN MATHEMATICS

*Lynda Ginsburg, Ph.D.*
*Center for Mathematics, Science and Computer Education,*
*Rutgers University*

Ginsburg said she is a math educator and the goal of her presentation is to provide a broad description of numeracy from a math education perspective.

Historically, in the United States, numeracy has been subsumed under literacy. For example, the National Assessment of Adult Literacy includes numeracy, and the West Virginia Department of Education defines literacy as "the ability to read, write, and speak in English, and compute and solve problems at levels of proficiency" (West Virginia Department of Education,

2013). Addressing numeracy as a separate issue from literacy is important, she said, because the issues are quite different.

Numeracy is different from school math. Ginsburg quoted Robert Orrill as saying that unlike math, "numeracy does not so much lead upward in an ascending pursuit of abstraction as it moves outward toward an ever-rich engagement with life's diverse contexts and situations" (Orrill, 2001, p. xviii). The difference is that in mathematics, the problems become more and more abstract. One math concept is the building block that leads to another. Numeracy, however, is applying mathematical reasoning and knowledge in increasingly diverse situations for different purposes.

The term "numeracy" was initially conceptualized in England and its use is relatively recent in this country, Ginsburg said. One of the earlier definitions of numeracy includes the concept of "at-homeness" with numbers and an ability to use math skills, which enable an individual to cope with practical mathematical demands of everyday life. A second definition includes having some appreciation and understanding of information that is presented in terms of numbers. Ginsburg believes this is where the medical field intersects with numeracy. Health and medical information is often presented in mathematical terms, graphs, charts, tables, and references to percentage increase and decrease. Often the concept of percentage increase and decrease is difficult for people to understand, even those within the health care field.

A different definition used in Australia explains that numeracy is a critical awareness that builds bridges between math and the real world and all its diversity. No particular level of mathematics is associated with this concept of numeracy. An engineer must be numerate, but so must a primary school child, a parent, a car driver, or a gardener. Numeracy is based on the different contexts in which each individual functions.

One final definition comes from an American, Lynn Steen, and lists five dimensions of numeracy:

- Practical, for use in everyday life;
- Civic, to understand and engage in public policy issues;
- Professional, to provide skills necessary for employment;
- Recreational, to understand games, sports, and lotteries; and
- Cultural, to be a part of the community and understand cultural context (Steen, 1997, p. xxii).

Ginsburg paraphrased Diana Coben (2000), saying that numeracy is an individual's ability to use his or her judgment about whether to use math in a situation, what math to use, how to use it, and what degree of accuracy is appropriate. An individual who is out shopping does not want to get to the cash register without enough money. This concern requires keeping track of the cost of the purchases, but the running total does not have to be exact. In fact, in that particular situation, it makes sense to round up because there will be tax or the shopper may have made an error. Making these kinds of decisions about what makes sense in each situation is the key to being numerate.

The components of numeracy, according to Ginsburg, include (1) context or purpose, (2) mathematical content, and (3) cognitive and affective processes (Ginsburg et al., 2006). When considering numeracy, it is important to think about the context or the purpose for the use of numeracy. This can be for further learning or, more importantly, for tasks in the workplace, the family, or the community. The mathematical content that goes into numeracy can include numbers, operations, patterns, functions, algebra, measurement, understanding measurement, and, for some contexts, shape, and also the use of data, statistics, and probability.

Finally, there are the cognitive and affective processes. Ginsburg cited a National Research Council report titled *Adding It Up* that defined these processes as the skills necessary to use math proficiently (NRC, 2001). First, a conceptual understanding of the mathematical ideas that are integrated and functional is necessary. A second necessity is reasoning, which is the ability to think logically about the relationships across ideas or within or between ideas and situations. Third is strategic competence, or having the ability to formulate problems and use appropriate strategies to solve them. Fourth is procedural fluency, which is the ability to do the calculations needed to solve the problem. Fifth, and perhaps most importantly according to Ginsburg, is a *productive disposition*, or the willingness to engage and use math skills to persevere in solving a problem as opposed to giving up. This process may face particular challenges in the United States as the focus of adult education interest has long tended to be on adult literacy rather than across literacy, numeracy, and language as is the case in other countries. Therefore, in American culture it is acceptable to say, "I cannot do math" and "Nobody in my family can do math," as if low numeracy skills are somehow genetic. While it is acceptable for people to say, "I cannot do math," it is not culturally acceptable for people to say, "I cannot read."

In the context of the workplace, a number of studies have shown the extent to which math skills are necessary and useful (FitzSimons, 2005; Hoyles et al., 2001; Marr and Hagston, 2007; Masingila, 1994; Smith, 2002; Zevenbergen and Zevenbergen, 2009). Ginsburg noted that it was interesting how often these skills were evident in work that is not generally considered to be mathematical, such as the work of supermarket employees, plumbers, or carpet layers. Across all of these workplace situations, the numeracy is deeply embedded in the context. What is done and how it is done depends on where numeracy happens and the purpose of the activity. People do things differently in different contexts for different purposes.

Often the numeracy is invisible. If people are asked if they use math in their jobs they will often say no, said Ginsburg, yet if their activities are analyzed, math is at least a part of what they do. These skills are often considered to be "common sense" by workers and not thought of as math skills. Math is often considered to exist only in a school context, with rigid rules and right or wrong answers. However, in the workplace, people develop their own solutions to problems, doing what makes sense to them in ways that make sense to them, Ginsburg said.

Sometimes the math is hidden by technology. For example, often bank employees inform customers about interest rates and securities, yet the employees do not know how the math calculations work because they never see them. The technology performs the calculations. In addition, some procedures become devoid of mathematical meaning in practice. Ginsburg related an anecdote in which she visited a construction site in Trenton where workers were renovating an old brownstone. The workers encountered problems with some beams they were installing and decided to measure the diagonals to determine if the outer walls were of equal length and perpendicular. When asked why they would measure the diagonals, the workers could not explain why, only that it was the way to tell if everything was going to line up correctly. The workers did not know the concepts involved, but they knew the procedure. There are many such examples from daily life.

Community-based numeracy involves interpreting information presented in the community, such as in the media. Ginsburg and Gal (1997) conducted a study in which they asked people to read an article in *USA Today* about a test that claimed to detect cancer in 90 percent of cases. Then they asked people to interpret that number. The results varied, with some people showing a good understanding of the proportional nature of percentages and others who were unable to do so. Importantly, said Ginsburg, it was not always easy to tell which individuals did not understand the number until follow-up questions were asked.

Another example of numeracy within the community comes from the Philadelphia public schools. Due to budget constraints, teachers were recently asked to take a 13 percent decrease in salary. Perhaps teachers would be offered a 13 percent increase once the fiscal crisis was over. Would this be fair to the teachers? This is more complicated than it appears at first, Ginsburg said, and people need to be able to figure out if they will come out even in this scenario.

Family and personal numeracy include things like shopping, cooking, and health-related decisions that are part of everyday activities. For example, Ginsburg said, an individual who is dieting needs to figure out three-quarters of two-thirds of a cup of cottage cheese. This can be calculated using the methods taught in school math class, but often people will figure out their own ways of solving problems, and those methods are valid if the solutions are correct. Shopping decisions are another example of family or personal numeracy, Ginsburg added. The store Bed Bath & Beyond sends out two types of coupons. Is it better to get "$5 off a purchase of $15" or "20% off of one single item"? Which coupon is better? The answer depends on the total cost and number of items purchased.

Given how vital numeracy is to everyday life, it is important to understand what Americans know about numeracy. The International Adult Literacy Survey included numeracy under the title of *quantitative literacy*, Ginsburg said. Quantitative literacy was defined by the survey as "the knowledge and skills required to apply arithmetic operations, either alone or sequentially, to numbers embedded in printed materials" (OECD, 2000, p. x). Of course, not all numbers come in printed material.

In the last two versions of the survey (1992 and 2003), the majority of Americans' quantitative literacy scores were in the lowest two levels, Below Basic and Basic. Forty-three percent of Americans scored in Below Basic or Basic levels for prose literacy, 34 percent for document literacy, and 55 percent for quantitative literacy, indicating that Americans demonstrated greatest weakness in the mathematical assessment, Ginsburg said.

The International Life Skills Survey, which contains a richer idea of numeracy because it includes how people manage situations and solve problems in a real context, involves responding to information about mathematical ideas. The information may not be in text, but rather involve a skill such as reading a gas gauge and making a decision based on that information, Ginsburg said. This requires the activation of a range of enabling knowledge, behaviors, and processes. This assessment was used in an adult education program study. The scores were expected to be relatively low because the respondents were adult education students in a high school equivalency program. Ginsburg noted that even taking that context into account, math skills were weaker than prose literacy skills.

Ginsburg also cited the General Educational Development test passing rates from 2012. Ninety percent passed the test overall, but only 80 percent passed the math portion (GED Testing Service, 2013). This illustrates that people across the board are weakest in math. At the community college level, the pass rate for all developmental math courses is 30 percent (Bailey, 2009). Overall, Ginsburg said, Americans are weak in math.

Ginsburg reiterated that numeracy can require counting, quantifying, computing, solving problems, and having a clearly right or wrong answer. It can also involve making sense of verbal, pictorial, or text-based messages based on quantitative data, without having to manipulate numbers, but just interpreting them. Numeracy can also mean finding and considering multiple pieces of information to determine a course of action, often without clear, correct answers. Ginsburg concluded by saying that these are the kinds of situations that arise in everyday life where numeracy is about solving a problem or making a decision, and always with a purpose and within a context.

## NUMERACY AND THE AFFORDABLE CARE ACT: OPPORTUNITIES AND CHALLENGES

*Ellen Peters, Ph.D.*
*Department of Psychology, Ohio State University*

In her presentation, Peters provided an overview of the roundtable commissioned paper that she wrote with two colleagues, Louise Meilleur and Mary Kate Tompkins (see Appendix A). She began by explaining why numeracy is important within the context of the Patient Protection and Affordable Care Act (ACA). Numbers are ubiquitous in health decisions, she said, whether determining the number of pills somebody takes, deciding what time of day to take those pills, or choosing among different treatment options based on risks and benefits. Numbers instruct, inform, and give meaning to information about health plans, medications, and treatments. But, Peters noted, not all people are able to understand and use numbers effectively when making health decisions. Even highly educated people, those with undergraduate and graduate degrees, are not necessarily numerate. Numeracy and education are related, but they are not synonymous with one another.

People who are innumerate tend to understand less numeric information; however, low numeracy skills are not just about comprehension of numeric information. People who are less numerate use numeric and non-numeric information in ways that are different from the more numerate. Innumeracy influences comprehension, but it also influences the use of information, Peters explained. When careful choices are made to present information in an evidence-based manner, these choices can lessen the effects of numeracy skill levels on how people understand and use information.

The first question is, "What does research show regarding people's numeracy skill levels?" Americans have limited numeracy skills, and disparities exist in those skills. People who are less numerate are more likely to be female, to be older, to be less educated, and to have lower income. According to Peters, some of these disparities are related to whether an individual currently has health insurance. This is important in the context of the ACA because the people who are going to have greater access to the health system because of the ACA are those people who do not already have health insurance, Peters said.

Numeracy can be measured in many ways, both objective and subjective. Peters focused on the results from the National Assessment of Adult Literacy (NAAL). That assessment estimated the proportion of Americans who fell into four quantitative literacy, or numeracy, performance levels.

Within the NAAL, an estimated 22 percent of the American population falls into a Below Basic level of quantitative performance, Peters said. She added that means that 22 percent of the U.S. population can do fairly simple number operations, such as locate numbers in a text, and perform simple quantitative operations such as addition if they are told that it is addition or it can be easily inferred from the situation. She noted that another third have somewhat more advanced basic quantitative literacy skills, and then another third have intermediate skills that allow them to locate less familiar quantitative information and use that information to solve problems. But, Peters said, only 13 percent of the population is considered proficient in numeracy. That means that 87 percent of the U.S. population cannot solve a problem where they are asked to calculate the yearly cost of life insurance using a table that gives the cost per month for each $1,000 of coverage.

As the first task in preparing the commissioned paper, Peters and her colleagues estimated the numeracy skill levels in the uninsured population. To do so, they examined two datasets. First, the NAAL provides numeracy levels by education and by population levels. U.S. Census data provide information on very similar education levels with health insurance status. Using these two datasets, of course, Peters said, the datasets do not align perfectly, but using both gives an idea of the relative numeracy levels between those people who currently have health insurance versus those people who do not but are likely to obtain it through the ACA.

Table 2-1 provides the results of the analysis. Peters estimated that 29 percent of the uninsured would fall in the Below Basic level of numeracy. That means they would be able to locate numbers in tables, for example, and perform simple operations. But they would not have the skills to perform operations at the higher levels. The uninsured would be less likely than the currently insured to be at the proficient level of numeracy.

As a result, numeracy issues are likely going to be more prevalent in the currently uninsured population that will gain access to insurance through the ACA. This means that health care providers are going to be faced with a different population of patients and consumers in comparison with the currently insured population. Whether providers will be prepared is a question because effective communication is different among people who are less numerate compared to people who are more numerate, Peters said.

In addition, numeracy issues may increase when people are in poor health. Being a patient may reduce deliberative capacity and the ability to think about numbers in particular. Stress may also reduce deliberative

**TABLE 2-1** Key Abilities and Estimated Proportion of Adults at Each Level of Quantitative Literacy

| Quantitative Literacy Level | Percentage of Adults in Each Level (National Assessment of Adult Literacy [NAAL] findings) | Estimated Percentage of Uninsured Adults in Each | Estimated Percentage of Insured Adults in Each | Key Abilities Associated with Level (NAAL) |
|---|---|---|---|---|
| Below Basic | 22% | 29% | 18% | Locating numbers and using them to perform simple quantitative operations (primarily addition) when the mathematical information is very concrete and familiar |
| Basic | 33% | 33% | 32% | Locating easily identifiable quantitative information and using it to solve simple, one-step problems when the arithmetic operation is specified or easily inferred |
| Intermediate | 33% | 29% | 35% | Locating less familiar quantitative information and using it to solve problems when the arithmetic operation is not specified or easily inferred |
| Proficient | 13% | 9% | 15% | Locating more abstract quantitative information and using it to solve multistep problems when the arithmetic operations are not easily inferred and the problems are more complex |
| Total U.S. population | 101% | 100% | 100% | |

SOURCE: Peters, 2013.

capacity. Patients are often under emotional stress and are overwhelmed by the quantity of information they are receiving about treatment options or regimens. Often patients are under time pressure because the decision must be made in the physician's office. According to dual-process theories in judgment and decision making, Peters said, this means that patient populations who are sick may not understand and use numbers as well in decision making, and they may rely on emotional sources of information that are easier for them to process. Little research exists on the topic, but it raises the question of whether current numeracy estimates, from the NAAL, for example, overestimate the skills of patient populations when they are sick.

The second task of the commissioned paper was to examine the numeracy skills necessary to perform a variety of tasks in the context of health and health care. To accomplish this task, Peters' team separated numeracy skills into two groups. The first group is called education-based numeracy skills, a concept discussed by Apter et al. (2008). These skills consist of knowledge about mathematical content and procedures. Within the education-based numeracy skills, Apter and colleagues identified a hierarchy of numeracy skills that are required to make health decisions. The skills range from very basic tasks, such as locating a number in a table or adding up premium costs, to skills that are somewhat more difficult, such as computational skills or working with frequencies and probabilities. Analytical skills are considered more difficult than computational skills in this hierarchy of numeracy skills. Statistical skills, which are often required for understanding the inherent randomness of life and the role of risk in making health decisions, are considered among the hardest of these skills.

Peters referenced an Agency for Healthcare Research and Quality report by Berkman et al. (2011) that concluded that having a theoretical basis to interventions made for more effective interventions to reduce health disparities. She explained that within the field of psychology of judgment and decision making, there is the idea that numeracy may exert its influence on health decisions and, through the making of health decisions, numeracy may ultimately influence health outcomes (Peters, 2012; Reyna et al., 2004). These emergent decision-based numeracy skills are psychological mechanisms that people have to go through in order to understand and use numbers. Some of these may seem very basic, yet there are differences based on numeracy. People who are highly numerate are actually more likely to seek out numeric information rather than avoiding it. It is not merely putting information in front of people and seeing if they understand it. It is about whether they will find the information for themselves.

Even if patients are given the information, there is the question of whether they will look at it because numeric information is usually given in the context of a great deal of other information, Peters said. People who are highly numerate are more likely to focus on numeric information, whereas people who are less numerate are more likely to look elsewhere. People who are more numerate also are more likely to ignore irrelevant information or less relevant information on a page. People who are more numerate also are more likely to recall numeric information, which can be important for issues such as medication adherence. There is a great deal of numeric information that must be remembered to facilitate health decision making and health behaviors.

People who are highly numerate tend to be more sensitive to numeric information, whereas people who are less numerate tend to be more sensitive to non-numeric and often emotional sources of information, such as what they have heard from friends and neighbors. The ability of the highly numerate to be more sensitive to numeric information may be due to a particular psychological mechanism, Peters explained. People who are highly numerate seem to derive more affective meaning from numeric information; that is, they are better able to interpret numbers within the context of the decision to be made. They are better able to tell not just that the number is 9 percent, but how good or bad this 9 percent is for them within the context of the decision. Research has shown that if an individual does not have a feel for the goodness or badness of a number, he or she is less likely to use it in judgments and decisions. Part of that greater sensitivity to numeric information that the highly numerate show may be due to their ability to derive meaning from numeric information and from comparisons of numbers, Peters said.

Table 2-2 displays the education- and decision-based skills required for some health decisions. The first column contains the quantitative literacy, or numeracy, level that was estimated for the uninsured population. The second column is a NAAL item that reflects that level of numeracy and the third column is a similar task required in health care decision making. The fourth is a breakdown of the skill categories necessary to the task.

The first example task, comparing and calculating the differences among the premiums of different health plans, falls into the Below Basic numeracy skill level. Peters and her colleagues estimated that about 29 percent of the uninsured population would possess Below Basic skill levels, meaning that most of the population and those with higher level skills would be able to complete this task. Peters stressed that not everyone will be able to complete the task, however. She noted that those who fall within the Below Basic category vary in their actual numeric abilities. She had conducted other studies that showed that about 7 to 9 percent of people who range from ages 18 to 64 were not even able to find very basic information in tables and charts.

Peters noted that in 2008 she coauthored a paper (Greene et al., 2008) that detailed the results of a study in which people looked at two different

**TABLE 2-2** Comparison of Tasks Based on Skill Level for Health Care Decisions

| Quantitative Literacy (Numeracy) Level | National Assessment of Adult Literacy (NAAL) Item | Example Task: Health Plan Selection | Skill Categories (Education-based, Decision-based) |
|---|---|---|---|
| Below Basic (29% of uninsured population; most of uninsured can do this) | Calculate the price difference between two appliances, using information in a table that includes price and other information about the appliances. | Compare and calculate the difference between monthly premiums of two plans. | Basic; Analytical Information Seeking; Attention |
| Intermediate (29% of uninsured population; 62% of uninsured likely cannot do this) | Determine what time a person can take a prescription medication, based on information on the prescription drug label that relates timing of medication to eating. | "The patient forgot to take this medicine before lunch at 12 noon. What is the earliest time he can take it in the afternoon? GARFIELD, Robert M. Dr. LUBIN, Michael DOXYCYCLINE 100MG Take one tablet on an empty stomach 1 hour before a meal or 2 to 3 hours after a meal unless otherwise directed by your doctor." | Basic; Analytical Information Seeking; Attention; Memory (if time of last meal was not provided) |
| Proficient (9% of uninsured population; 91% of uninsured likely cannot do this) | Determine the number of units of flooring required to cover the floor in a room, when the area of the room is not evenly divisible by the units in which the flooring is sold. | Diabetes management: understanding glucose meter readings, interpreting sliding-scale regimes, titrating oral medications or insulin, adjusting insulin for carbohydrate content. (Note: This example is much more complex than any of the NAAL examples used.) | Basic Computation; Analytical Information Seeking; Attention; Memory; Information Sensitivity; Affective Meaning |

SOURCE: Peters, 2013.

health insurance plans—one that was a new concept for health insurance and one that was a more traditional health plan. The authors asked the study participants a number of comprehension questions about these two plans, Peters said. They found that most people understood which plan had the lowest monthly premium, but only about one-third could identify which plan was better if the patient needed a great deal of care. The authors estimated that the more difficult task of determining which was the more valuable insurance is at an intermediate level of proficiency.

Understanding medication and treatment instructions is another example of health care information that requires an intermediate level of proficiency, Peters said, citing an item from the NAAL that addresses health care directly and also requires an intermediate level of proficiency. The example is that of a patient who forgot to take medication and must figure out the earliest time he can take the next dose. Participants are given information about the time of the patient's last meal and the instructions on the medication bottle. Because about 29 percent of the uninsured population falls within the intermediate numeracy level, according to Peters' estimate, approximately 62 percent of this population would not be able to answer this item correctly. These individuals may lack the ability to determine the correct way to adjust medication if a dose has been skipped.

Peters said her team estimates that about 9 percent of the uninsured will be at the proficient level, meaning that 91 percent of the uninsured population will not be able to do the tasks at that level. Some of the tasks involved in, for example, diabetes management or other chronic disease management require these higher level skills.

The final question addressed in the commissioned paper is how providers can best communicate with individuals with lower numeracy skills. The proportion of the uninsured population who will be able to correctly perform different kinds of tasks will often depend on how that information is presented. Health materials can require greater numeracy skills or fewer numeracy skills to read and understand, depending on how the materials are formatted. Peters listed some of her recommended strategies for communicating with less numerate individuals:

1.  Provide numeric information as opposed to not providing it. Numbers inform, educate, and give meaning to information. In short, numbers matter.
2.  Reduce the cognitive effort that is required. Individuals who are less numerate are less comfortable dealing with numbers. Giving careful attention to the ways in which numeric information is presented is critical among this population. A variety of techniques can help those who are less numerate to better understand and use important health information.

3. Provide evaluative meaning for numeric information. This can occur through the use of symbols or interpretive labels. This is particularly helpful when the numeric information is unfamiliar.
4. Draw attention to important information. People who are less numerate are less likely to attend to numeric information, even when it is provided. There are techniques that can be used to draw attention to important numeric information.
5. Set up appropriate systems to assist consumers and patients. One of the most important parts of these appropriate systems is to determine the goal of the communication. Once a goal has been identified, then the provider or health educator can use the evidence base to find the best way to communicate to the less numerate population to meet that goal.

Health decisions and health behaviors involve a great deal of numeric information either explicitly or implicitly, Peters said.

Peters concluded by saying that the average numeracy skills in the population brought into the health insurance and health care systems by the ACA are likely to be lower than that of the current population in those systems. It is also important to note that they likely have more limited knowledge and experience in health settings. As a result, how information is presented may matter as much as what information is presented, particularly to these less numerate populations. Peters also stressed that communication strategies should be evidence based and that various strategies should be tested within this population to determine which are the most effective.

## DISCUSSION

*Moderator: Paul Schyve*

Rima Rudd, roundtable member, commented that the example used in Peters' presentation of comparing and contrasting two different health plan options is considered by educators and developers of assessment tests to be a very sophisticated task that is well beyond basic skills. The hierarchy of skill levels begins with the simplest task of finding one piece of information, then moves on to the more difficult task of finding two similar pieces of information. A process like comparison and contrast is considered to be a high-level skill. Rudd said she thinks that most people at basic-level numeracy would have difficulty accomplishing that task with accuracy and consistency.

Peters responded that a great deal depends on context. People's abilities will depend on whether they are given information in short form without other irrelevant information around it or if they are trying to locate multiple pieces of information within a complex format, as will occur with the health insurance exchanges. Tasks can differ in difficulty depending on how they are presented.

Patrick McGarry, roundtable member, commented that some patients distrust numbers generally and asked Peters if she took into account the qualitative nature of numeracy. Peters answered that as far as she is aware there is little research on the qualitative aspect of numeracy. She said that there is evidence that people who are less numerate tend to trust numbers less within the health context and may be more likely to avoid numbers and not focus on numbers even when presented with them. This can make a difference in how much people interact with numeric information or avoid it in making judgments or decisions.

McGarry followed up by quoting Mark Twain as saying there are "lies, damn lies, and statistics" and noting that many people believe this. He said it is a challenge that practitioners face in discussing numbers with their patients. Peters responded that in her view it depends a great deal on how the numbers are presented. For example, she noted that evidence shows that people perceive less risk of adverse events from prescription drugs and are more willing to take the drugs if they are provided information on risk numerically as opposed to some other way. This appears to be the case across numeracy levels. Peters said it also depends on the quality of communication. If the information is communicated in a very complex way, then the patient may be less likely to trust it because he or she does not understand it. Context is always an important issue in numeracy. Ginsburg added that this challenge is related to the fact that people often perceive information according to their biases. She said it is important to be aware of this and remember that people may be responding according to emotion rather than the data that are being given to them. Schyve added that he thought this was an example of confirmation bias, where an individual is more likely to believe something that fits his or her current beliefs. He said this is true in narrative literacy, but also in terms of numbers. Peters responded that some people simply do not trust numbers and do not trust information in the health system. She noted that there can be large cultural differences in the way people respond to information. She thinks, however, that some of that distrust can be alleviated if more careful attention is paid to how information is presented.

Ruth Parker, roundtable member, asked the speakers, "If you could do one thing to have an impact on patient protection and affordability and public health within the Affordable Care Act, what would it be? What are the opportunities in the current environment that could help people in the new system?" Peters said she would have default options available for people through the health insurance exchanges that best suit their needs, but it is difficult to estimate individual health care needs. The amount of information presented to the consumer on the exchanges can be overwhelming, even for the highly literate and numerate. This can create a highly stressful situation that will prompt strong emotional reactions and cause people to think they cannot cope. She would also reduce the number of choices that people have available through the exchange because having too many choices is also overwhelming and reduces people's ability to make good choices.

Ginsburg agreed that fewer choices and a default option on the exchanges would help the process become more manageable for most people. She would also like knowledgeable people to be available to walk consumers through their options and help them make the best choices for their situation. Peters added that the experience from Medicare Part D suggests that a number of people will choose their plan based primarily on monthly premium cost. Yet that is not always the best option, particularly for people who require a great deal of health care. Parker responded by saying that she believed those answers helped reframe the discussion from what cannot be done by the consumers to what can be done by the exchanges to help the consumers. Peters added that she believed that studying the challenges of a situation leads to better solutions.

Roundtable member Wilma Alvarado-Little asked how the presenters envisioned the role of the health insurance exchange navigators (those people who will help consumers) in alleviating some of the problems caused by low numeracy and how they would empower navigators to address these issues. Peters said it is important for the navigators to have the communication skills necessary to understand what is important to the consumer, whether that is lower monthly costs or avoiding a potential large lump sum cost. The health insurance exchanges can be thought of as information about different health insurance packages and the navigator is trying to uncover the goals of the consumer in order to guide them to the most appropriate product. The navigator should understand some of the evidence base for effective communication, she said. It is tempting to think that all that is necessary is to provide accurate information and people will make their decisions based on that information. Yet just providing information is often not enough, particularly for people who are less numerate. Tools that allow navigators to quickly display options in a way that individuals who are less numerate are more likely to understand would be a valuable resource for navigators to have.

Roundtable member Steven Rush commented that the issues of health literacy and numeracy go beyond the acquisition of health insurance. Once people have been brought into the system, how can information be presented that allows them to make appropriate decisions about their health care? He added that the role of stress in decision making is very important and that even highly numerate people can be innumerate in crisis situations. Ginsburg agreed that the big decisions in the short term are about choosing and enrolling in a plan, but over the long term interacting and negotiating with insurance companies may be the larger challenge. She noted that it will be important for patients to be able to advocate for themselves and family members and enlist provider support at times to support them in their interactions with insurance companies. This may be an empowerment issue as well as a literacy and numeracy issue.

Rush responded that high numeracy to a certain extent brings empowerment. He wondered what would be the best way to provide numeric-based information to people when they are already in a health plan so that they can communicate better with their physicians and understand their treatment options. Peters said this is a huge topic and there are a number of strategies that can be applied, depending on the specific health situation and the goals of communication within that health situation. First it is important to ask, "What is the most important information for the patient to understand and use?" Once the most important information is determined, then delete the less important information, Peters said. Some techniques involve informing the consumer or patient and helping him or her understand the numbers and their meaning, while other techniques are persuasive. For example, warning graphics on cigarette packages are meant to be informative, but also persuasive. Different strategies are chosen depending on the goal of the communication. Peters added that this brings up the topic of educating health care providers about communication strategies, which is often an overlooked strategy in improving health. The people providing the information must know the best way to communicate in different situations.

Schyve commented that there are ethical questions contained in the suggestions to limit information and choices for consumers, and that different situations would call for different solutions. For example, public policy makers may decide there would be a limited number of insurance plans offered through the exchanges. Regarding the question of choice in treatment, however, it may be unethical to withhold some information even if it makes the options more difficult for the patient to understand. This may mean that it is up to the provider to spend more time helping the person understand his or her options. There could still be a default choice, but all available information must be given to the patient.

Benard Dreyer, roundtable member, asked about the relative importance of written versus verbal communication when communicating numeric information. Peters answered that there has not been much research on verbal communication of numeric information; most of the research has been done on written communication. That raises some questions because most health care providers communicate verbally. Peters thinks numeric

information would be better communicated verbally with written supporting materials, but there is no research to support it. It is an important
research question, but it is often overlooked because it is difficult to study.

Dreyer then asked what strategies work best when dealing with information that is so complex that it demands numeric proficiency from the
patient. For example, Dreyer said, diabetes care requires a high level of
numeracy that is difficult to simplify. Peters said it is likely there are studies
concerning numeracy and diabetes, but she is not aware of them. She said it
is helpful to give people concrete indicators of some action. For example, if
the blood sugar level hits a certain point, then a specific action is required.
This gives people something to remember or write down and have available to use as a guide. Helping people understand the goodness or badness
of the numbers involved in their care is also important. For example, a
patient given a range of numbers may not understand that a certain number
in front of him or her is in that range. The provider must help the patient
understand what numbers are in the range and whether they are good or
bad. Ginsburg added that from a mathematical education perspective, multiple representations of a concept help people understand and learn math. It
would be helpful for patients struggling to make sense of new information
to be given the information in different ways. Patients can receive verbal
instructions along with tables and written information that they can study
or graphical information that they can review with the provider.

Cindy Brach, roundtable member, noted that people with low numeracy skills would likely have a great deal of insight into this situation because
they must develop coping strategies. For example, Brach said she once
spoke with an adult learner who told her that although he was a truck
driver, he could not read a map. To cope with this situation he would stop
at diners along his route and chat with people to get directions, which he
would write down and stick to his windshield. It would be worthwhile to
ask patients the best way to help them learn and remember what they need
to know.

Robert Logan from the National Library of Medicine (NLM) said
that both presenters spoke about research showing that increasing a person's interest, engagement, involvement, and eventual numeracy capability
could result from providing tailored materials for them and other strategic interventions. Both presenters also mentioned that an opportunistic,
contextual transformation occurs based on a person's role. For example,
a website called patientslikeme.com illustrates that people with no medical training can develop an impressive knowledge of medicine in the right
circumstances. Logan asked if there was any research literature on how
to take advantage of that opportunity with a patient and help the patient
overcome any literacy or numeracy issues in that context. Peters answered
that she was unaware of any research explicitly on the transformation pro-

cess. Some studies look at people's ability to choose high-quality hospitals given a variety of information. Researchers found that people who are more numerate are more likely to choose high-quality hospitals, and people who are more health literate according to reading levels are also more likely to choose high-quality hospitals. Yet women, who tend to be less numerate, are more likely than men to choose high-quality hospitals. This is likely because women are more likely to have more experience within health settings. Women are more likely than men to be responsible for family health care and as a result have developed additional skills. Peters added that there has been a great deal of research on the patient activation process, which is a related topic. She recommended the work of Judith Hibbard of the University of Oregon. Hibbard's research focuses on taking patients from one level of activation to another.

## IS NUMERACY MORE DIFFICULT WITH POOR HEALTH?: EVIDENCE, EXPERIENCE, AND POSSIBILITIES

*Terry Davis, Ph.D.*
*Professor of Medicine and Pediatrics,*
*Louisiana State University Health Sciences Center, Shreveport*

Does poor health affect numeracy? The answer, Davis said, is probably, but she could find no studies in the literature on the topic. However, many studies indicate that poor health and chronic disease can impact cognition, but none were specifically related to numeracy.

Davis spoke about her personal experience as a patient, noting that since she has been on the faculty of a medical college for 30 years and has done extensive research into health literacy, she should have proficient health literacy skills. At age 60, Davis was very healthy and had never missed a day of work because of illness. She took no prescription or over-the-counter (OTC) medications and was unfamiliar with the benefits and restrictions of her health insurance plan. A visit to the cardiologist changed everything when she learned that she would need open-heart surgery to correct a heart defect. Although Davis found her diagnosis confusing and overwhelming, she was able to conduct some online research and consult with friends to help her make decisions about her care. She did not, however, ask her employer or health insurer about possible restrictions on providers or hospitals.

Davis chose the best place for her procedure based on quality of care considerations without taking into account that the provider was not part of her insurer's network so, unbeknownst to her, it entailed a 30 percent copay. The admission and preoperative process was very well organized and the surgeon spent time with Davis and her family answering questions. The discharge process after the surgery was a much more disorienting and rushed experience. The discharge nurse listed Davis' medications very rapidly and seemed annoyed when asked to write down the indication for each medication. Davis said she felt lost and overwhelmed and remembered hoping that her husband was better able to understand the instructions than she was.

Davis said she found the names of the various prescription medications difficult to remember and pronounce. In addition, there are differences between brand names and generic names for the same medication, and it can be embarrassing for patients to mispronounce medication names in front of health care providers. She felt unsure of the medication instructions and she was far from home and her usual pharmacy. Her husband filled her prescriptions. The pharmacist did not give any oral instructions and Davis' husband did not ask questions. The first night out of the hospital, Davis was unsure if she had been given all of her medication for that day when at the hospital. She called the hospital where the procedure was performed, but her file had already been deleted from the computer so the nurse was not able to tell her what medication she had been given at discharge. Davis said she felt vulnerable and overwhelmed by the situation.

The instructions on Davis' medications varied and were written in a convoluted manner. For example, the label of one medication read, "Take 1 tab (10 mg) by mouth once daily except Tuesday and Thursday; 1 & ½ tabs (15 mg) once daily on Tuesday and Thursday," which she found very confusing and hard to read. Davis' medication list was extensive and she was often not told why she had been prescribed certain medications or how long she would be taking them. In addition, she was told to take some medications "as needed," but was not given any instructions on what symptoms would indicate need.

Davis also spoke of her experience with pain medications. She was discharged from the hospital with OTC and prescription pain medications, but not told whether to take them concurrently. In addition, the prescription medications also contained acetaminophen, a common ingredient in many OTC medications that can be dangerous in high doses. Davis was never warned about her acetaminophen dosage or instructed to be aware of how much she was taking. After conducting research with colleagues, Davis said she found that the majority of consumers do not read OTC medication instructions. In addition, people develop their own schematics for taking OTC medication based on what they have always done or what others around them have done, but not based on the instructions provided with the medication.

Davis said additional medications for conditions unrelated to her heart were added to her drug regimen. The dietary instructions related to these medications were often confusing and difficult to follow. For example, the instructions for an osteoporosis medication to be taken once a week read, "Take with 8 ounces of water at least 30 minutes before first food or beverage of the day. Don't lie down for 30 minutes." Davis said she found this very difficult to work into her routine, so she devised a modified regimen of her own. This was particularly difficult to do when traveling, she said, so she did not take this medication when she traveled. Many medications look alike and can be difficult to tell apart. This is especially worrisome when using medication organizers. For some medications it may not matter if a patient accidentally takes a double dose, thinking he or she is taking two different medications, Davis said, but for other medicines that can be dangerous. When the prescription changes from a brand name to a generic, the size, shape, and color of the pill also may change. This can be very confusing for the patient.

Davis noted that she and many others must also face the well-meaning suggestions of friends and family members regarding their illness and treatment plan. Patients may be encouraged to stop taking some medications based on a news story or website, or encouraged to supplement their medications with alternative medicines. She cautioned that clinicians must be aware of these external influences and their impact on a plan of care.

System redesign does not have to be complex, Davis said. It can be as simple as responding to Joint Commission recommendations and implementing teach-back methods before and after a procedure. Providers can simplify medication instructions and solve numerical problems for the patient. Emerging research suggests that a simplified, clearer medication label can affect understanding and adherence.

Other issues concern medicine and numeracy, Davis said. For example, does having alcohol with dinner affect one's ability to take medication at night? Being distracted or sleep deprived might also affect the ability to follow medication instructions. Feeling stress or being away from home may also have an impact. Finally, the medications themselves may affect numeric skills and cognition.

Davis said she learned several important lessons about following a complex drug regimen. First, hospital discharge is the beginning of a process that requires time and energy to manage. Second, patients must understand the treatment plan and be able to engage in problem solving to make it work. This includes learning to embed medicines into everyday life and manage disruptions to the routine. Patients must plan ahead and develop confidence in communicating with providers and insurance companies. Finally, Davis said, high literacy and assertiveness do not guarantee adequate health literacy.

Insurance was another area that tests even the strongest numeracy skills, Davis said. It is difficult to find answers to questions on which policy to choose and what various policies cover. Bills from providers and statement of benefit documents from insurance companies can be hard to read and understand. Even employees of insurance companies often have a difficult time explaining the statement of benefits to consumers. It is difficult to know which source of information is trustworthy, Davis added. Insurance companies sell many types of policies, and it is hard to understand the differences or know which one is best for an individual.

Davis cited an article in *The New York Times* by Gina Kolata (2013) about trying to determine the cost of a medical procedure. Kolata was attempting to find the cost of a vaginal delivery for her daughter, who was uninsured. In the article, Kolata quotes Dr. Uwe Reinhardt from the University of Pennsylvania as saying that hospitals are not required to tell patients the cost of a procedure upfront and often hide that information until they send a bill. Private insurers claim they let patients know what out-of-pocket costs are likely to be, Davis said, but when Kolata checked with one insurer's website and called the company hotline, she could not find out any information on cost. In the article the question is asked, "How can people make good choices about health care if they cannot find out about cost or quality?"

Davis said if she could effect change in the health care system, she would provide clear and accessible information on cost and quality and have informed and friendly navigators available by phone to personally assist with medicine and insurance questions. She would do away with the phone trees, long holds, and suggestions to call another department that she endured. It took Davis 13 months to settle the insurance for her surgery. Davis also said she would mandate patient-centered hospital discharge instructions; universal and easy-to-read and -navigate instructions on all prescription and OTC bottles; and what she calls an "Apple store" approach to buying and using insurance. Davis noted that when she goes into an Apple store the cost is obvious and the staff are objective and patient when explaining the technology to customers, who may be overwhelmed or do not know what they need.

Davis encouraged those at the workshop to form an action plan to address some of these issues. She noted that health literacy is the interaction between the skills and abilities of the patient and the demands of the system, and that providers need to be prepared to address the demands of the system. This could take the form of standardizing prescription and OTC labels and medicine guides to make them easier to see, navigate, understand, and follow.

Davis concluded by reminding the audience that technology is a tool that does not replace a nice, knowledgeable person. As many in the room know, Davis said, health is personal.

## DISCUSSION

### Moderator: Paul Schyve

Benard Dreyer, roundtable member, commented on the issue of patients using the appearance of a medication as a tool to understand what they are taking. In his practice the doctors have been experimenting with different asthma action plans and have found that many families use the color of the inhaler to determine which medication it is. Dreyer said it would be helpful if inhaler labeling or packaging were standardized so that all albuterol is one color and all steroids are another color. He asked if there was a way to use the appearance of medications to overcome low health literacy and numeracy. Davis replied that she thinks people respond to color. She related the story of buying a new printer and being guided by colors to set it up—the blue goes with the blue and the green goes with the green. Technology companies use this method to help people who are not experts to use their products correctly, Davis said.

Robert Logan from the NLM commented that the NLM was completing work on a website that contains high-quality images of pills to help consumers identify medications. The website is operational as of summer 2013 and serves as an important resource for patients.[1]

Rima Rudd, roundtable member, commented that one of the issues around pills and numeracy is that instinctively people assume that small is small and big is big and big is more powerful than small. When patients move from a brand name drug to a generic drug, often the pill sizes change and there are times when the pill size for a larger dosage is smaller than that of a smaller dosage. This is very difficult for people to manage and leads to medication mistakes. Rudd said that size is a system issue that must be addressed along with color and name. Names of drugs are often chosen because of the sound, Rudd said. For example, drugs that are meant for heart-related conditions have strong sounds in them such as Ks and Ts and other powerful consonants. Drugs that are meant to soothe and relax have soft sounds such as Ss, Cs, and Xs. This means that medications for similar conditions almost all sound the same making it very confusing for people to remember the name of their specific medication.

Kim Parson, roundtable member, commented that the research on the patient-centered label is very interesting and she would like to understand more about it. She noted that in terms of adherence one of the challenges is helping people understand what to take and when. Parson agreed that health care is personal and added that the even the same procedure is dif-

---

[1] The website, known as Pillbox, is available at http://pillbox.nlm.nih.gov (accessed October, 29, 2013).

ferent for every patient. Davis responded that presentations later in the day would give more information about the current state of the research. She said that researchers are working toward understanding how to help people with their medications but there is no one solution that will help everyone. No matter how patient centered the final label is or how unique the pill shape, some people will still need personal help.

Susan Pisano, roundtable member, commented that although Davis had many advantages she still felt overwhelmed by the complexity of her care regimen and the system. She asked if there was anybody or anything that was helpful in guiding Davis through the system. Davis answered that there was nothing within the system that was helpful but that she relied on outside friends and contacts to give her advice. Pisano asked about the day before Davis' procedure, which had gone well, and what it was about that day that worked well and was helpful. Davis answered that the care before the procedure was organized and convenient. Everything was in one place and was organized with the patient in mind.

Margaret Loveland, roundtable member, commented that speaking from a pharmaceutical industry point of view she understands the frustration of the different look and size of generic medication. For example, the day after Singulair, a medication manufactured by Merck, went off patent there were 20 generics approved that came onto the market. Each one looked a little different and it is easy to see how patients get confused. The active ingredient in generic medication is nearly always the same or at least very similar, but the inactive ingredients are different. Davis asked if the pharmaceutical companies are trying to make the names easier. Loveland answered that it is difficult to get new names. There are few one- or two-syllable names and they are all gone, so the names continue to get more complex.

Loveland also said that she believes that for people coming into the health care system via the ACA there will have to be better communication about why they should have health insurance. The costs of health care and reasons for insurance will have to be explained in a way that people can understand.

## REFERENCES

Apter, A., M. Paasche-Orlow, J. Remillard, I. Bennett, E. Ben-Joseph, R. Batista, J. Hyde, and R. Rudd. 2008. Numeracy and communication with patients: They are counting on us. *Journal of General Internal Medicine* 23(12):2117-2124.
Bailey, T. 2009. *Rethinking developmental education in community college*, CCRC Brief. Community College Research Center, Teachers College, Columbia University. http://ccrc.tc.columbia.edu/media/k2/attachments/rethinking-developmental-education-in-community-college-brief.pdf (accessed October 30, 2013).

Berkman, N. D., S. L. Sheridan, K. E. Donahue, D. J. Halpern, A. Viera, K. Crotty, A. Holland, M. Brasure, K. N. Lohr, E. Harden, E. Tant, I. Wallace, and M. Viswanathan. 2011. *Health literacy interventions and outcomes: An updated systematic review.* Evidence Report/Technology Assessment No. 199. (Prepared by RTI International–University of North Carolina Evidence-based Practice Center under contract No. 290-2007-10056-I.) AHRQ Pub. No. 11-E006. Rockville, MD: Agency for Healthcare Research and Quality.

Coben, D. 2000. Mathematics or common sense? Researching invisible mathematics through adults' "mathematics life histories." In *Perspectives on adults learning mathematics: Research and practice*, edited by D. Coben, J. O'Donoghue, and G. E. FitzSimons. Dordrecht, The Netherlands: Kluwer Academic Publishers. Pp. 53-66.

FitzSimons, G. E. 2005. Numeracy and Australian workplaces: Findings and implications. *Australian Senior Mathematics Journal* 19(2):14-40.

GED Testing Service. 2013. *2012 annual statistical report on the GED Test*, GED Testing Service. http://www.gedtestingservice.com/uploads/files/8d4558324628dfcf1011dc738acca6eb.pdf (accessed October 30, 2013).

Ginsburg, L., and I. Gal. 1997. Uncovering the knowledge adult learners bring to class. In *Adults returning to study mathematics*, edited by G. E. FitzSimons. Adelaide, Australia: Australian Association of Mathematics Teachers. Pp. 55-61.

Ginsburg, L., M. Manly, and M. J. Schmitt. 2006. *Components of numeracy.* Occasional paper. Cambridge, MA: Harvard Graduate School of Education, National Center for the Study of Adult Learning and Literacy. http://www.ncsall.net/fileadmin/resources/research/op_numeracy.pdf (accessed October 30, 2013).

Greene, J., E. Peters, C. K. Mertz, and J. H. Hibbard. 2008. Comprehension and choice of a consumer-directed health plan: An experimental study. *American Journal of Managed Care* 14(6):369-376.

Hoyles, C., R. Noss, and S. Pozzi. 2001. Proportional reasoning in nursing practice. *Journal for Research in Mathematics Education* 32(1):4-27.

Kolata, G. 2013. What does birth cost?: Hard to tell. *New York Times*, July 8.

Marr, B., and J. Hagston. 2007. *Thinking beyond numbers: Learning numeracy for the future workplace.* Adelaide, Australia: National Centre for Vocational Education Research.

Masingila, J. O. 1994. Mathematics practice in carpet laying. *Anthropology & Education Quarterly* 25(4):430-462.

NRC (National Research Council). 2001. *Adding it up: Helping children learn mathematics*, edited by J. Kilpatrick, J. Swafford, and B. Findell. Mathematics Learning Study Committee, Center for Education, Division of Behavioral and Social Sciences and Education. Washington, DC: National Academy Press.

OECD (Organisation for Economic Co-operation and Development). 2000. *Literacy in the information age: Final report of the International Adult Literacy Survey.* http//www.oecd.org/edu/skills-beyond-school/41529765.pdf (accessed May 14, 2014).

Orrill, R. 2001. Preface. *Mathematics and democracy: The case for quantitative literacy*, edited by L. Steen. The National Council on Education and the Disciplines: The Woodrow Wilson National Fellowship Foundation. http://www.maa.org/sites/default/files/pdf/QL/MathAndDemocracy.pdf (accessed October 29, 2013).

Peters, E. 2012. Beyond comprehension: The role of numeracy in judgments and decisions. *Current Directions in Psychological Science* 21(1):31-35.

Peters, E. 2013. *Numeracy and the Affordable Care Act: Opportunities and challenges.* Presentation at the Institute of Medicine Workshop on Health Literacy and Numeracy, Washington, DC, July 18.

Reyna, V. F. 2004. How people make decisions that involve risk: A dual-processes approach. *Current Directions in Psychological Science* 13:60-66.

Smith, J. P. 2002. Everyday mathematical activity in automobile production work. In *Everyday and academic mathematics in the classroom*, edited by M. E. Brenner and J. N. Moschkovich. Reston, VA: National Council of Teachers of Mathematics. Pp. 111-130.

Steen, L. A., ed. 1997. *Why numbers count: Quantitative literacy for tomorrow's America.* New York: The College Board. P. xxii.

West Virginia Department of Education. 2013. *Adult literacy defined.* https://wvde.state.wv.us/abe/definingstatus.htm (accessed October 29, 2013).

Zevenbergen, R., and K. Zevenbergen. 2009. The numeracies of boatbuilding: New numeracies shaped by workplace technologies. *International Journal of Science and Mathematics Education* 7:183-206.

# 3

# Numeracy Demands, Assumptions, and Challenges for Consumers

The presentations from this panel address the numeracy demands on patients and consumers made by the health care and health insurance systems. The first speaker was Lynn Quincy, who spoke about the challenges people face when choosing a health insurance plan. Quincy is a senior policy analyst for the Consumers Union, the policy and action arm of *Consumer Reports*. The second speaker on the panel was Andrea Apter, a professor of medicine at the University of Pennsylvania. Her presentation discussed the role of numeracy in understanding health care and medical treatment.

## OVERCOMING CONSUMER BARRIERS TO SHOPPING FOR HEALTH INSURANCE

*Lynn Quincy, M.S.*
*Senior Policy Analyst, Consumers Union*

Consumers Union carried out consumer testing of the new health insurance disclosure requirements in the Patient Protection and Affordable Care Act (ACA), Quincy said. In that process they learned a great deal about how people are struggling with this issue and the challenges for people trying to make sense of this information. Her presentation is about the numeracy issues involved in shopping for health plans, Quincy said.

People dread shopping for health insurance because they do not understand the product, she explained. This is an important barrier for people who are beginning the process of purchasing insurance. Yet they realize there are important health and financial implications for them and their families, which increases the stress associated with purchasing health insurance. In addition, consumer testing showed that people have little trust in health insurance companies, another source of stress in the process.

Consumers Union research showed that the primary reason why people cannot determine which plan is best for them is that they are confused by the cost-sharing terms, Quincy said. There are a number of numeracy components to this issue for consumers. Consumers are not sure of the definitions of terms such as "deductible," "out-of-pocket limit," and "annual benefit limit." These are complex concepts on their own, but in the context of individual health insurance plans, the consumer also needs to understand how they work together. For example, does the copay count toward the out-of-pocket limit? The consumer needs to know the answers to questions like this to be able to choose the best plan for his or her situation. Quincy said this task is nearly impossible for consumers at the point of shopping for a plan.

She illustrated the point by giving an example of the cost-sharing term "coinsurance." There are three distinct issues surrounding coinsurance for most consumers. First, understanding the meaning of the term and its implications is difficult for some consumers. Many are confused about who is paying the indicated percentage, particularly if that number is at the extremes such as zero percent and 10 percent or 90 percent and 100 percent. Even when this information is provided, the consumer has a difficult time understanding. Second, how is a percentage calculated? This is a very challenging, if not impossible, task for many consumers. Quincy recalled one consumer who could not calculate 70 percent of $1,000. The consumer said that it was "about half." She continued to answer that the percentage represented half even when the number was changed. Calculating and applying percentages were beyond her math skill level. Finally, to what number does the percentage apply? Even those who were proficient with percentages could not answer this question because the number is never given. The percentage applies to the "allowed amount," but this amount is never shared with the consumer. Thus it is impossible for the consumer to know his or her obligation in advance. As a result, even the consumers with the highest numeracy skills cannot make well-informed choices.

Quincy said that for her this raises the question of how things can be made better for the consumer. Her first recommendation is to conduct consumer testing to learn what the challenges are for consumers operating in this environment. Consumer testing provides information for the path forward.

After learning what the barriers and challenges are for consumers, Quincy recommended the following steps:

- First, improve the product as much as possible.
- Second, improve communication about the product.
- Third, educate and activate consumers.

In the context of health insurance, improving the product means simplifying it for consumers. The ACA accomplishes some of this, Quincy said, by standardizing the out-of-pocket limit so consumers do not need to be aware of exceptions, and the term means the same thing across plans. Standardizing products is very helpful because there are fewer things for consumers to track. Some states, such as Massachusetts, have gone further and standardized the benefit design for a given tier or service. Consumers do not have to compare factors such as copays and coinsurance because they are identical, so they can focus on premiums and quality measures.

Communication about the product can be improved in several important ways, Quincy said. Consumers will always use cognitive shortcuts to make decisions; proactively developing cognitive shortcuts is one way to help them make informed choices. For example, showing the consumers the estimated cost for common health care needs such as having a baby, treating diabetes for a year, or treating breast cancer can have an enormous impact on their perception of both health care and health insurance. Further showing what an insurance plan will pay versus what the consumer will pay is also a powerful tool because it does the math and eliminates some of the confusion about benefits and consumer obligations. Consumers Union research detailing who will pay was very important to consumers, who often thought of insurance as prepaid health care and did not realize that the insurance company would bear some of the cost. Presenting information in ways that are clearer to the consumer can help overcome some of the numeracy barriers and remind people of the value of insurance. Another example is the plan comparisons associated with the *Consumers' Checkbook Guide to Health Plans for Federal Employees and Annuitants*,[1] which allow individuals to compare various components of health plans and customize an estimate of average yearly cost. Such information empowers consumers to make better decisions.

Quincy concluded by saying she believes that the challenges can be overcome and that the research and knowledge exist to give consumers better tools that will allow them to shop for health insurance with confidence. This can be accomplished through consumer testing and application of that knowledge.

---

[1] The *Consumers' Checkbook Guide to Health Plans for Federal Employees and Annuitants* is an online tool that allows federal employees and retirees to compare health insurance plans offered under the Federal Employees Health Benefits Program.

## NUMERACY IN HEALTH CARE: A CLINICIAN'S PERSPECTIVE

*Andrea J. Apter, M.D., M.Sc., M.A.*
*Professor of Medicine, University of Pennsylvania*

Apter said that she approaches numeracy in health care and health decision making from the perspective of the clinician. Many procedures are involved in numeracy. The hierarchy of numeracy skills is organized into overlapping categories by level of difficulty (Golbeck et al., 2005). This hierarchy is important because it provides the complete picture of numeracy concepts.

Basic skills, the first category in the hierarchy, concern the ability to identify and read numbers. The next category involves computational skills, meaning the ability to do counting and arithmetic procedures. Next in the hierarchy is the category of the more difficult analytical skills: inference, estimation, proportion, percentage, frequencies, and basic graphs. Apter believes that analytical skills play a large role in health care and in clinicians' directions to patients because these skills enable patients to interpret information. The final category in the hierarchy is statistical skills, including probability, statistics, error, and risk. Statistical skills allow patients to compare things and understand probability, which are important concepts in health care. Patients encounter all of the concepts involved in numeracy when they receive care, follow treatment plans, and pay for medical care.

Much of chronic disease care is based on informing patients about prevention and risk, which requires an understanding of statistics and probability, Apter said. A number of tasks are involved in managing a chronic disease, and numeracy skills are required for all of them (see Box 3-1). First,

---

**BOX 3-1**
**Some Tasks Involved in Managing a Chronic Disease**

- Understand the disease
- Participate in the development of a management plan
- Follow the management plan
- Monitor symptoms
- Use measurement devices and record readings
- Take medicine as prescribed
- Note changes in status
- Present the story and exchange information with the clinician

SOURCE: Apter, 2013.

patients must understand the disease itself, along with the symptoms. This often entails understanding frequency, trends, and decreases and increases in severity, all of which are numerical concepts. Apter added that patients must also participate in the development of a chronic disease management plan, which is often complicated and involves a variety of numeracy skills. Such skills are also needed to follow the management plan; for example, patients must monitor their symptoms. To do this they may have to use measurement devices and record and track results, such as peak flow meter readings in asthma care or blood glucose measurements in diabetes management. They also need to be able to note changes in their health status and make judgments about whether those changes are significant. Most importantly, Apter said, patients must present their history to the clinician and be able to participate in a conversation about their care.

Apter showed an example of an action plan from the National Heart, Lung, and Blood Institute that illustrates the complexities that patients may face (see Figure 3-1). The action plan is based on the concept of a traffic light—green means the patient is doing well, yellow means that symptoms are getting worse, and red means the patient must take action to improve their symptoms. The action plan requires that medications and dosages be recorded. In following this plan, patients may need to understand frequencies, trends, and variation, and some analytical skills are required. Patients are also asked to measure and record their best peak flow on the action plan. They also must understand what is 80 percent of their best peak flow and the range of 79 to 50 percent of their best peak flow. These measurements are indicators for patients to use in tracking the severity of their asthma symptoms. Clinicians may also ask patients to graph the results of these measurements taken over time. Yet patients may not have the skills to understand and participate in this action plan.

Another typical situation that tests patients' numeracy skills, Apter said, is discharge instructions from a hospital or emergency room. For example, a man who was hospitalized with an exacerbation of chronic bronchitis was given a pill bottle containing prednisone tablets when discharged. Each tablet was 5 milligrams. The man was told to take 30 milligrams, requiring him to solve the problem of how many tablets to take. This is not an easy problem to solve for many people, particularly in a stressful situation. Another example is of cancer patients who are confronted with the standard gamble problem. The standard gamble concept is intended to help patients and clinicians discuss preferences in the context of cancer diagnosis and treatment. A person is asked to give preferences for treatment by stating whether he or she would rather remain in a state of ill health for a period of time or undergo a medical intervention, which has a chance of either restoring perfect health or killing the patient. The concept of the time trade-off is another example of a problem that a patient is often expected

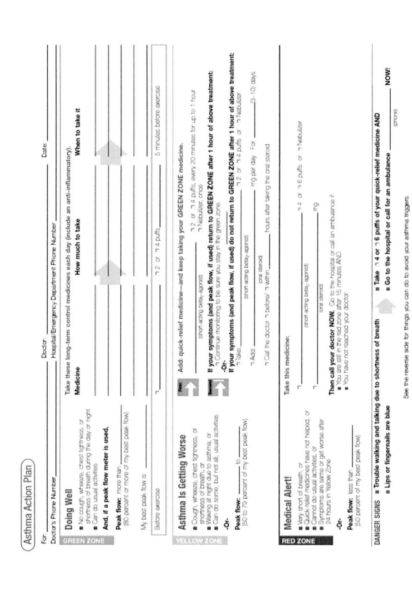

**FIGURE 3-1** Asthma Action Plan from the National Heart, Lung, and Blood Institute.
SOURCE: Apter, 2013.

to understand and solve. It is important to remember, Apter emphasized, that this is all in the context that more than 50 percent of Americans have no more than basic numeracy skills. It can be difficult for many people to understand these concepts and use them in making health care decisions.

To conduct research into the numeracy skills of asthma patients and whether it affected their asthma care, Apter and colleagues developed the Asthma Numeracy Questionnaire, a four-question survey on common concepts in the national asthma guidelines, and administered the survey to patients in English or Spanish (see Box 3-2) (Apter et al., 2006). The first question was the prednisone dosage question given previously. When asked the question of how many 5 milligram tablets to take to equal 30 milligrams of prednisone, 84 percent of patients with moderate to severe asthma recruited from a clinic answered correctly. That means, however, that 16 percent did not understand those instructions. The next question was about risk and percentage. Steroids are often prescribed in asthma care and there is a risk that a patient could get osteoporosis from taking steroids for a prolonged time. Patients were asked to give an explanation of a 1 percent chance of developing osteoporosis. Only 38 percent of patients could correctly explain the concept of 1 percent; most did not understand.

The final two questions covered peak flow meter readings, often used in asthma management, Apter explained. First, patients were asked to determine 50 percent of their personal best peak flow meter reading if their personal best is 400 liters. Nearly three-quarters of patients were able to answer correctly, but that means that more than a quarter of patients were not. Second, patients were asked a more complicated peak flow question using percentages to determine a range of readings that indicated a "Worry Zone." Only 20 percent of patients were able to correctly identify the range of readings that equaled 50 to 80 percent of the given peak flow reading, Apter said.

When the survey results were compared with the participants' scores on the Short Test of Functional Health Literacy in Adults (STOFHLA), there was only a moderate correlation between the two. Apter said there could be a number of reasons there is not greater correlation. It could be that numeracy is very different from reading comprehension, or that the test characteristics are different, or that the numeracy questions were in the context of asthma and asked of asthma patients. A more important result of the research was the finding that low scores on the numeracy questions were associated with more emergency department visits and hospitalizations for asthma. This association did not appear to be present with the STOFHLA.

Apter said that as she monitored patients over time as part of another research project, a higher numeracy score was associated with better asthma control and quality of life. The research showed that lower numeracy skills were associated with poorer health. This is an important link, Apter said,

**BOX 3-2**
**Asthma Numeracy Questionnaire (ANQ)**

**ANQ Question 1**

Here are some examples of statements or questions patients might hear in a doctor's office.

1. Your doctor asks you to take 30 mg of prednisone every day for a week. The pharmacist gives you a bottle of 5 mg tablets. How many pills should you take each day?

**ANQ Question 2**

If a patient has a 1% chance of developing osteoporosis or bone loss, that means:

a. Out of 1,000 patients, one will develop bone loss
b. Out of 100 patients, one will develop bone loss
c. Out of 10 patients, one will develop bone loss
d. Out of 5 patients, one will develop bone loss
e. The patient will develop bone loss
f. The patient will never develop bone loss

**ANQ Question 3**

You have a peak flow meter.
Your Danger or Red Zone is 50% of your best reading.
Your best reading is 400 L/min. What is your Danger Zone?

**ANQ Question 4**

You are told the Green Zone (the OK zone) is a reading between 80% and 100% of your best reading. Your Worry Zone is between 50% and 80% of your best reading. Your best reading is 400 L/min. When are your readings in the Worry Zone?

a. Between 300 and 400 L/min
b. Between 200 and 320 L/min
c. Between 200 and 300 L/min
d. Between 240 and 320 L/min
e. Between 100 and 300 L/min

SOURCE: Adapted from Apter, 2013.

and leads to the question of what should be done to improve low numeracy skills. There are things that could be done at a societal level, such as ensuring adequate and equal educational opportunities for all, and at the patient level, such as confirming patient understanding. Apter said she would focus on what clinicians can do to overcome the negative consequences of low numeracy skills.

Apter suggested that clinicians should focus their efforts in two areas—first to decrease the demand on the patients and second to increase clinician communication skills. Apter and colleagues developed a matrix (see Figure 3-2) as a guide to decreasing the numerical demand on patients. The columns list numerical concepts arranged in order of difficulty, from simple operations such as recognizing numbers to complex operations such as determining risk according to the classifications described by Golbeck and colleagues (2005). The rows display the level of mastery required in

| Numeracy element | Level of Patient Mastery Required (demand on patient) | | |
|---|---|---|---|
| | Describe | Interpret | Decision Making |
| Reading numbers, counting, telling time | | | |
| Arithmetic operations | | | |
| Estimation of size, trend | | | |
| Frequency | | | |
| Percentage | | | |
| Problem-solving and inferring the mathematical concepts to be applied | | | |
| Logic | | | |
| Reading tables | | | |
| Reading graphs | | | |
| Reading maps | | | |
| Estimation of error, uncertainty, variability | | | |
| Relative versus absolute | | | |
| Risk (cumulative, relative, conditional) | | | |

FIGURE 3-2 A matrix for simplifying patient–provider communication.
SOURCE: Apter, 2013.

the communication. Descriptive information is the easiest to understand, followed by interpretation and then, finally, decision making.

Apter hypothesized that determining where a piece of information fits into the matrix and then working to simplify the information so that it would move up and to the left on the matrix would make the information easier for the patient to understand. For example, using the issue of the number of 5 milligram prednisone tablets to take to achieve a 30 milligram dose, the clinician could instead instruct the patient to take six pills in the morning, thereby moving the communication up and to the left on the matrix. The style and content of the instruction would move from the "problem-solving" row to the "reading numbers" row. Instructions given in this way would place lower numerical demands on the patient. Another example of simplifying the communication is to tell a patient to lose a certain number of pounds rather than a percentage of body weight. This would move the communication up and to the left on the matrix. For tasks such as monitoring information over time, which includes understanding trends, the clinician may be able to simplify the communication by graphing the information for the patient.

Developing different ways of framing the information is another way to decrease the demands on the patient, Apter said. For example, comparing the 5 milligram tablets of prednisone to nickels may be a helpful way to give context to the patient. However, it is important that the framing be appropriate. Both patients and physicians will interpret information differently depending on how it is stated. People may make different decisions if told they have a 70 percent chance of death if given certain chemotherapy versus a 30 percent chance of living. Visual aids such as graphs and charts can also help decrease the demands on the patient, but it is important to use the appropriate graph at the appropriate time.

Apter said that clinicians can also focus on improving their communication skills. She cited an article by Peters and colleagues (2007) that stressed the need to remove extraneous information and give patients only the most essential information. Using plain language when communicating with patients is also very important, Apter said, as well as engaging in "teach-back" with patients to confirm their understanding of what has been said. A patient advocate can also be helpful in patient–provider communication. A patient advocate is someone close to the patient, such as a family member, who can accompany the patient to a medical visit and serve as a way to check that the patient and provider are communicating effectively. Although teach-back and discussions with an advocate can be time consuming for the clinician, there are ways to delegate some of the process to other staff in the practice. Another literacy skill that is becoming increasingly important is electronic literacy. Technological resources can be daunting for many people, but they also have great potential for providing yet another format for presenting health information, particularly numerical information.

In closing, Apter said there are significant unrecognized numeracy demands for adults with chronic diseases. Poor numeracy is associated with poor health outcomes, and limited numeracy can impair the ability to communicate and understand health information and to participate in shared decision making. It is essential to equalize and enhance educational opportunities, but clinicians must also understand and account for limited educational opportunities and limited numeracy in patients to ensure adequate access to health care and effective communication, Apter said.

## DISCUSSION

### *Moderator: Paul Schyve*

Steven Rush, roundtable member, agreed with Apter's assertion that electronic literacy is important and becoming more so because people are increasingly expected to conduct health-related tasks online. Rush noted that Quincy had done research on health insurance literacy and asked if she could give a brief overview of her work on that topic. Quincy said she had presented some of the same research at an earlier Institute of Medicine workshop (IOM, 2012) and at that time had noted a need for a better way to measure health insurance literacy. There are good measures for health literacy, but these measures do not capture the challenges in purchasing health insurance. Since that 2011 meeting, the American Institutes for Research (AIR) has begun working on measures of health insurance literacy; however, numeracy may not be broken out as a separate measure. Quincy said she would prefer a scoring system that could identify which component of the score was related to numeracy, literacy, and other skills.

Rush commented that AIR is using an approach similar to that taken by the National Assessment of Adult Literacy (NAAL). Furthermore, some of the AIR work is related to the uniform glossary produced by the U.S. Department of Health and Human Services and the U.S. Department of Labor, which attempted to simplify terms such as copay, deductible, and coinsurance. Rush said that the Consumers Union also had produced a good usability test for the definitions of terms produced by the National Association of Insurance Commissioners. These definitions were ultimately moved into the uniform glossary.

Quincy replied that the glossary was produced as a tool to accompany a standardized method of explaining insurance policies and net summaries of benefits and coverage. The glossary is written in plain language and examples are included in the text. Consumer testing showed, however, that because it is a standalone product and is not context sensitive, most people said they were unlikely to seek out the glossary if they were having trouble understanding an insurance policy or explanation of benefits. The glossary can be very helpful, Quincy concluded, but it cannot be assumed that consumers will always seek out helpful information. It may be necessary to provide the information to the consumer in the policy to ensure that it is reaching them.

Rima Rudd, roundtable member, expressed a cautionary note about emphasizing measuring people's skills or lack of skills. Skill levels are already known through the national assessment tools. She noted that measuring a problem again and again does not help solve the problem and that she is encouraged by an emphasis on actionable items and testing possible solutions to the problem of low numeracy.

Benard Dreyer, roundtable member, asked what Quincy had learned through her research about the confusion surrounding the difference in cost between in-network and out-of-network providers. Quincy answered that the consumer testing conducted by her organization did not delve too deeply into that topic. She noted, however, that based on other research and the experience of advocates, the difference between being in network and out of network is a source of confusion for consumers. The primary source of confusion is a lack of understanding of the financial implications of being in network versus out of network. People understand that going out of network will be more expensive, but it is difficult to determine how much more expensive. One component of the ACA that has yet to be implemented is to work to improve measures of network adequacy. A number of people are working on that and it will likely include ways to capture the influence of time, distance, geography, and other measures of whether a network meets consumer needs. Quincy believes that measures of network adequacy could be taken further and include not only how broad or narrow a network of physicians is, but also how financially accessible that network is and whether the physicians have the capacity to accept new patients. These are dimensions of a network that consumers need to know.

Dreyer commented that his medical practice has been trying to design a better asthma action plan. He said the example from Apter's presentation is confusing for parents, particularly for those who do not speak English or have low literacy skills. His practice has made the decision to eliminate peak flow measurements from its asthma action plan because it is so confusing. Originally he was against this idea, but its elimination has helped parents understand the plan more easily by reducing the cognitive load. Apter agreed and said she used it in the presentation because it is a good example of something that is commonly used, but difficult for patients to understand.

Patrick McGarry, roundtable member, noted the American Heart Association's Know Your Numbers campaign, which asks people to track their blood sugar, blood pressure, blood cholesterol, and other various health measures. He asked Apter if she was aware of any research that examines whether tracking and knowing measures like those improves an individual's health. Apter answered that she was not aware of any research into the efficacy of tracking such information. Quincy pointed out that many times a consumer information tool is created and distributed without any follow-up testing of its effectiveness.

Roundtable member Linda Harris commented that a key target population for health insurance under the ACA is healthy young men. She asked if there is any research on whether health literacy or numeracy may be a challenge with this group. Quincy said the research does not address that topic specifically, but that encouraging people to obtain health insurance was a goal of her organization as well. Quincy said that from her understanding of the available research, she believes that there is a motivational challenge for young men. They are not necessarily motivated by arguments related to health, but may be motivated by arguments related to the financial consequences of not having insurance coverage.

Susan Pisano, roundtable member, asked if Apter has any experience using her decision matrix with medical students, pharmacy students, or nursing students and, if so, how it was received. Apter replied that she has discussed the concepts with residents and medical students, who received it respectfully, but she has not shown them the matrix. Rudd commented that she has used the matrix many times with public health students and that they have been enthusiastic about it because it is a useful tool. Rudd said she did not know whether any of them continued to use it in practice, but it has been received positively in an educational setting.

Cindy Brach, another member of the roundtable, expressed interest in removing nonessential information as one way of bridging the gap between abilities and demands. She said that she and two colleagues, Michael Wolf and Sarah Shoemaker, have developed a patient education materials assessment tool, which is a tool that assesses whether materials are understandable and actionable. Brach asked if there are any strategies to help people who are writing and designing patient information materials to determine what is not essential. Apter said she does not know if there is formal guidance, but she thinks nothing can replace a conversation between a patient and a provider that discusses patient understanding and priorities. She noted that with regard to electronic health records, for example, there is a place in the after-visit summary for providing individualized information to the patient. This may become a critical way to communicate pertinent information to the patient as providers and patients become more accustomed to electronic records. This would, however, require educating both providers and patients in its use, Apter stressed.

Quincy said that on the health insurance side, the difficulty of deciding what information is essential and what is not is an important point. She said she does not know of any overarching strategy for making these judgments while designing materials, but well-designed consumer testing can reveal what is essential and what is not and guide the revision of materials.

Lindsey Robinson, roundtable member, asked if Apter knew of any asthma action plan that included information on the impact of asthma medications on oral health. Apter answered that oral health in general is not considered enough in medical education and medical treatment, and is not generally mentioned in asthma treatment. She added that this is an issue because oral health is important for overall health and quality of life. Robinson agreed and noted that she was aware of several cases where children had severe tooth decay caused in part by their asthma medications. The children's caregivers had not been made aware that these medications contribute to tooth decay. Apter said there is little in the research literature on the topic, although she has heard a number of anecdotes like Robinson's and formal research needs to be done.

Robinson asked Quincy if, in the course of her research on consumer understanding of health insurance, she had looked into consumer knowledge about dental insurance. Under the ACA many families will receive dental insurance for the first time, and it is confusing for both families and providers. Quincy said she has not engaged in research on dental insurance, but she is familiar with others' research. People want dental coverage as part of their health insurance. It is a motivating factor even for those who are young and healthy and not otherwise interested in health insurance. The implementation of the ACA with regard to dental insurance has been confusing because it is offered as a standalone policy, and there are a number of questions about whether purchasers are eligible for tax credits or if dental insurance alone fulfills the individual mandate. This will likely continue to be an area of confusion for consumers, Quincy said.

Roundtable member Margaret Loveland asked Apter what she meant during her presentation when she said that it is essential to equalize and enhance educational opportunities. Did she mean for children, consumers, or physicians? Apter said she was referring to educational opportunities in public schools. Her experience as a math teacher showed her that the math taught in schools, whether rich in resources or not, is not always the math people use in their daily lives. Apter said that research shows that health disparities are rooted in disparities in income and education.

Darren DeWalt, roundtable member, commented that Quincy is performing a vital task in helping consumers understand health insurance, but that it is frustrating that health insurance products seem to continually grow more complex. He believes this complexity is taxing everyone's resources and increasing the difficulty for consumers and those who are trying to help them. DeWalt added that he, like Brach, is interested in the question of how to determine which information is essential and which is not. For example, Quincy asked in her presentation whether consumers need to know the total cost of treating breast cancer or just the cost to the consumer. As an example from Apter's presentation, is it necessary for the patient to know the difference between a controlling medication versus a rescue medication for asthma? Perhaps, DeWalt said, the patient only needs to know that one is taken every day and one is only taken when symptoms appear.

DeWalt added that asking consumers and patients what information is meaningful to them is the only way to know. Quincy said the state and federal insurance exchanges operating under the ACA provide a good research opportunity because they each display and present information to the consumer a little differently. She added that in her coverage example, it was important for the consumer to know the total cost of breast cancer treatment because that knowledge provided motivation to buy insurance. The total cost versus the cost to consumer provided important contextual information. Apter noted that it is important to remember that not everybody needs a simple explanation, and the provider must tailor information to the individual patient. She added that, as a physician, she believes it is important for patients to know the differences in their medications.

Wilma Alvarado-Little, roundtable member, asked if there has been any discussion of whether providers could help patients determine whether a specialist is in network or out of network, for example, by reminding patients to check with their insurance companies when they receive a referral. Quincy replied that she has not seen any research on that topic, but that it might be a good idea to add a reminder to check on a provider's status on the referral slip. She did not think, however, that providers would want to take over that responsibility. Kim Parson, roundtable member, agreed that providers do not want to get into the details of a patient's health insurance. She noted that her company, Humana, proactively contacts policy holders who are referred to out-of-network providers to offer the opportunity to switch to an in-network provider. Alvarado-Little commented that patients often trust their provider more than anyone else and may not trust the insurance company. Quincy agreed that it is important that information come from a trusted source or consumers will not pay attention to it. Parson replied that insurance companies do not have the same relationship with a patient as a provider does, but that Humana finds it appropriate to provide that information to customers, and that the majority of the time the customer switches to an in-network provider.

Laurie Francis, roundtable member, commented that a patient-centered medical home and a team approach are necessary to accomplish everything that the presenters and roundtable members are discussing. There is not

enough time for a provider to handle treatment, prevention, patient education, and health insurance questions. Some of those things are better left
to advocates, health coaches, and nurses, among others. She asked if the
team approach is considered when working on how to best help patients.
Apter answered that a team approach can be useful, but has its challenges.
First, there may be no standard team for coordinating care of a chronic illness. Second, communication is a challenge across multiple providers and
practices.

Heidi Silver-Pacuilla from the U.S. Department of Education said she
was delighted that the roundtable had addressed the issue of adult numeracy and literacy. She informed the roundtable and the audience about a
new data source for research on the health literacy, numeracy, and digital
literacy skills of adults—an Organisation for Economic Co-operation and
Development study called the Program for International Adult Assessment
Skills and Competencies (PIAAC).[2] The study consists of nationally representative data from 24 countries in the first round and 9 more countries
in later iterations. The first sample is not as large as the NAAL sample,
but it will continue to grow as the study moves forward. The data will be
available for public use and a number of tools will be available to assist
researchers in analyzing the data. Silver-Pacuilla emphasized that people are
not stuck at low levels of literacy and numeracy. She added that involvement in their own and their families' health is an opportunity for people to
learn new skills and new concepts. Her experience has shown that as people
learn they become advocates for their families.

John Gardenier, audience member, commented that the presenters had
discussed numeracy with regard to medications and medical treatments,
but what about exercise, diet, and lifestyle? Don't patients need numeracy
and literacy skills to understand their physician's advice about those topics?
Quincy and Apter both agreed that better health habits should be promoted
systemwide.

Helen Osborne, audience member, said that after hearing the morning's
presentations, she was excited and enthusiastic about possible solutions to
the problem of low numeracy skills. She wondered if the challenges could
be reframed to fit with the Apple store analogy offered earlier by Terry
Davis. When health care tasks are deconstructed, everything relates to
problem solving and decision making, she said, and it is exciting to think
of new ways to approach these challenges.

Audience member Bill Elwood noted that many of the lessons learned
and challenges discussed by the morning's presenters point to the need for
basic research. What are the cognitive steps that people take when making

---

[2] More information about the PIAAC can be found at http://www.oecd.org/site/piaac/
surveyofadultskills.htm (accessed October 29, 2013).

decisions? How do people learn and increase their numeracy skills? Answering questions about these types of basic human processes can advance health literacy research and improve people's health.

Jessica Ancker, a presenter scheduled for the afternoon session, noted that much of the morning's presentations had been about costs and the difficulty of estimating medical costs. She drew the roundtable's attention to a website, Fairhealth.org, which provides publicly available information on the costs of various procedures. Quincy pointed out that Fairhealth.org allows consumers to look up the Current Procedural Terminology (CPT) code for a procedure and find the usual and customary charge or the Medicare charge for a specific area. This assumes, however, that an individual has the skills to locate the CPT code and use the website. In addition, Quincy said, most consumers lack the ability to build what is called an "episode," that is, to include all of the CPT codes involved in a procedure or medical treatment. The website also cannot answer the question of what a specific hospital will charge for a procedure, which is usually what the consumer needs to know, Quincy concluded.

## REFERENCES

Apter, A. J. 2013. *Numeracy in health care: A clinician's perspective.* Presentation at the Institute of Medicine Workshop on Health Literacy and Numeracy, Washington, DC, July 18.

Apter, A. J., J. Cheng, D. Small, I. M. Bennett, C. Albert, D. G. Fein, M. George, and S. Van Horne. 2006. Asthma numeracy skill and health literacy. *Journal of Asthma* 43(9):705-710.

Golbeck, A. L., C. R. Ahlers-Schmidt, A. M. Paschal, and S. E. Dismuke. 2005. A definition and operational framework for health numeracy. *American Journal of Preventive Medicine* 29(4):375-376.

IOM (Institute of Medicine). 2012. *Facilitating state health exchange communication through the use of health literate practices: Workshop summary.* Washington, DC: The National Academies Press.

Peters, E., N. Dieckmann, A. Dixon, J. H. Hibbard, and C. K. Mertz. 2007. Less is more in presenting quality information to consumers. *Medical Care Research and Review* 64(2): 169-190.

# 4

# Numeracy Demands, Assumptions, and Challenges for Communicators

The third panel presentations were from Marguerite Holloway, from the Columbia University Graduate School of Journalism, and Jessica Ancker, an assistant professor at the Center for Healthcare Informatics and Policy at Weill Cornell Medical College. Their presentations examined the role of the media in communicating health information to the public and the challenges faced by communicators in effectively communicating risk and uncertainty.

## NUMERACY AND HEALTH JOURNALISM

*Marguerite Holloway, M.S.*
*Columbia University Graduate School of Journalism*

Holloway said the issue of numeracy and health journalism is a vital one. A number of things can lead to confusion and mistakes in the coverage of science news, including misinterpretation of results, institutional spin, discarded caveats and context, time constraints, and the fixed beliefs of the audience. These problems are as familiar to audiences as they are to journalists. The issues of numeracy and medical reporting have been written about a great deal and there are excellent books, reports, and studies to consult, Holloway said.

Numeracy in science and medical reporting remains an issue of ongoing professional discussion and concern. In preparation for her talk, Holloway noted that she spoke with a manager at the Association of Healthcare

Journalists who confirmed that numeracy and improving health reporting remain areas of high priority for the organization and areas in which they frequently do training and outreach. Journalism, generally, not just in health and medical reporting, is relying increasingly on data analysis, numeracy, and statistical savvy. Holloway said that her presentation addresses the challenges posed to journalists by numbers in health reporting, strategies that journalists can or should use, and the ethical issues that can arise.

Holloway said she could find no definitive numbers on how many Americans get what proportion of their information about health from journalists. It is clear from responses to news stories that many people get and use health information presented by the media and that media outlets respond to consumer demand by presenting health stories, particularly on personal health. In this context getting the numbers wrong or creating hype has the potential to have significant consequences, Holloway said. People can make bad choices about care, treatments, or lifestyle, which can lead to poor decisions such as refusing vaccines for children. Media stories can give people false hope or great disappointment and no hope. For example, people can become desperate for a new cancer drug that they later learn is not available or has only been tested on animals or they can waste money on medications that are no different from cheaper ones already on the market. Holloway pointed out that media coverage can drive research and funding into areas that might not be as significant for public health as others and can cause people to lose trust in science and medicine.

Most journalists are aware of the impact their stories can have and take that responsibility seriously, Holloway said. Reporters face a number of challenges, however, some shared by society at large and others that are specific to the field of journalism. First is the baseline challenge that many, if not most, people have some trouble with numbers. If something can be numerically expressed, Holloway said, it carries with it a sense of authority and fact. As a result numbers are influential, and they can have long lives even if they are errors, being cited again and again and shaping public understanding of a topic. Yet although people respect numbers and attribute power to them, they want to engage with numbers as little as possible.

According to Holloway, this peculiar combination of skittishness and reverence becomes evident in the fact that numbers in media stories often exist side by side with basic mathematical mistakes. A 2012 examination of one daily newspaper found, for instance, that nearly half of the stories, a total of 536, published over the course of 1 month included or required some kind of mathematical information or calculation (Maier, 2012). The study also found that errors were prevalent in these and other stories. The author of the article identified 11 types of mistakes, including incorrect addition, misinterpretation of numbers, sensationalization using dramatic numbers, and unquestioning use of figures. Many errors were of elementary math, errors that common sense could easily catch, but few reporters or editors had turned their attention to the numbers. Basic prevalent attitudes toward math are one fundamental challenge, Holloway added.

A second major challenge is a lack of understanding of scale and scalability, Holloway said. Researchers such as Gail Jones at North Carolina State University have shown that appreciating scale is a key to scientific thinking. Problems of scale as it relates to dimension can extend to people's problems interpreting and contextualizing numerical health information. Numbers of cases or rates of disease are difficult to scale up or down in an accurate or meaningful way. A number can have one meaning or implication when considering an individual's personal circle of friends and acquaintances or community, and another with regard to the U.S. or global population. Few people are able to move fluidly up and down those scales to see the personal and the big picture accurately, Holloway said.

A third challenge relates to statistical thinking or understanding probabilities, ranges, risks, and ratios. This represents a mathematical skill or habit of mind that can be particularly challenging for the press and public alike. A 2002 study surveyed 165 journalists and found that 84 percent of the reporters, 96 of the respondents, had never been trained in understanding health statistics (Voss, 2002). The importance of correctly interpreting statistics and the difference it can make is captured in an essay written in 1985 by Stephen Jay Gould titled "The Median Isn't the Message," Holloway said (Gould, 1985). The essay is widely known and is very helpful in thinking about patients and numeracy. Gould writes of learning of his cancer diagnosis and reading in the medical literature that patients with this cancer have a median mortality of 8 months. He notes that most people would take this to mean that they had only 8 months to live. Gould writes that this conclusion must be avoided because it is untrue, and attitude matters a great deal in approaching serious illness. He goes on to explain that one must understand that variation is the reality and mean and median are abstractions. He wonders whether he might be in the groups of patients who will live longer than 8 months, which he learns he is. He then learns that the distribution is right skewed with a long tail and he may live years beyond the median, which he does. Holloway said that Gould explains the statistics so clearly that his essay is a model of how to explain commonly used statistical concepts in terms that are easily understood. The essay also provides a reconciliation of what Gould calls the unfortunate and invalid separation between heart and mind or feeling and intellect. As an example of this, Holloway said studies about public perception of climate change information illustrate the difference between the experiential processing system and the analytical processing system. The tension between these two ways of processing information is another challenge for reporters covering health.

Some challenges faced by reporters, however, are specific to journalism. Many media outlets are losing money and decreasing numbers of staff, and many reporters have to do more in less time, Holloway said. The profession has always been driven by deadlines and intense competition, but now reporters and writers in many places must be constantly producing content. There is often less time to be reflective and little incentive to wait to publish a story to analyze the numbers, the implications, and the context.

The academic journal culture is an additional challenge for the press. Holloway said that science, health, and medical information largely come from studies that are embargoed to build a "news peg" to create buzz and often revenue for the journals themselves. Daily journalists are embedded in a cycle that is nearly impossible to escape from while keeping pace with the competition. A reporter on a deadline often does not have the time to examine a number too closely and there is little opportunity to think historically under those conditions or take time to understand the information in context. This culture does not favor an appreciation of medicine or science as incremental and uncertain, and stories with too many caveats are not "newsy," Holloway said. In these conditions, most reporters do the best they can and set aside questions for more in-depth examination for longer stories or perhaps a trend story. These are more analytical reflective pieces where issues are examined more deeply and with nuance and where numeracy is handled in much better or clearer ways.

Holloway presented several strategies that journalists use or should use and that journalism students are taught. Some of the strategies are not specific to numeracy issues, but are generalizable ways of thinking about approaches to reporting on science, health, and medicine. Journalists should be familiar with various types of studies and their limitations, Holloway said. Reporters should not misrepresent or overinterpret the significance or implications of findings and should have a roster of basic questions to ask about any study. The reporting about how research works must be transparent and present the strengths and weaknesses of different types of studies. It should also look beyond the one study to reviews or meta-analyses that may have been done in the field. Journalists should find a statistician they can rely on and turn to for advice and guidance, Holloway said. As news organizations adapt to the new environment, there is more collaboration with statisticians and data experts in newsrooms. Holloway recommended that numbers be presented with transparency and in a variety of ways, and that journalists give both relative and absolute risk. According to Holloway this practice is not as routine as it should be; a review of 500 news stories in 2008 found that only 18 percent gave both relative and absolute risk (Schwitzer, 2008).

An example can be found in the review of a story about suicide rates by Paul Raeburn, who assesses the press coverage of science for the Knight

Science Journalism Tracker (Raeburn, 2013). The original story reported that the suicide rate had increased by 30 percent in those ages 35 to 64 between 1999 and 2010, from 13.7 deaths per 100,000 to 17.6 deaths per 100,000. As Raeburn notes in his review, but the original story failed to do, a 30 percent increase sounds large, but the absolute numbers are much smaller. The increase amounts to approximately 4 more people per 100,000 and suicide remains a rare event for this age group, occurring in much less than 1 percent.

Holloway noted that it is important that journalists maintain skepticism about the study and the numbers being reported. This can mean thinking about the history of a figure and not taking anything for granted. A good example of investigating a widely used statistic can be found in "How Long Can You Wait to Have a Baby?" in *The Atlantic*, which looks at the assumptions underlying fertility (Twenge, 2013). The author of the story noted that most sources reported that one-third of women between 35 and 39 would not be able to get pregnant within 1 year of trying and that women in their late 30s had a 30 percent chance of never having a child. After tracking down the source of these numbers, the author discovered that they are from an analysis of French birth records from between 1670 and 1830. The author notes that there are not many well-designed studies of female age and natural fertility that include women born in the 20th century, but those that do have different, and more optimistic, results.

Holloway said it is also important to blend the statistics and stories of people in a compelling way in order to capture both the data and the human experience. Many journalists do this beautifully when they have time and some space and support, she said. She added that journalists should repeat as often as possible that correlation is not causation.

Holloway concluded by noting that everyone tries to force information, including numbers, into the frame of the mental model they already have. It is difficult to absorb information that runs counter to expectations. When journalists tell stories of individual experience that are well supported by and help illustrate numerical data, the complexity and nuance of the issue can come to life. In this way numbers can have a transformative effect. Engaging with numbers, getting them right, understanding their implications, and then presenting them in the public realm is for the greater good and benefit for society.

## ISSUES AND CHALLENGES IN THE
## ERA OF SHARED DECISION MAKING:
## EXPLAINING RISK AND UNCERTAINTY

*Jessica S. Ancker, Ph.D., M.P.H.*
*Center for Healthcare Informatics and Policy,*
*Weill Cornell Medical College*

Ancker's presentation explored the ways in which numeracy issues relate to shared decision making and the concept of explaining risks and uncertainty. She began with an example of a patient decision that generated a number of headlines early in 2013, when Angelina Jolie publicly disclosed that she had tested positive for mutation at BRCA1 and chose a prophylactic bilateral mastectomy as a preventive measure. Jolie's decision received a great deal of attention because of her celebrity and the radical nature of her choice, Ancker said. It is instructive to examine the editorial Jolie wrote explaining her decision. In the editorial, Jolie discusses her family history of breast and ovarian cancer and her desire for more information, which led to seeking out the BRCA tests. When Jolie tested positive, she was given a lifetime risk of developing breast cancer of more than 80 percent, which is obviously very high. Jolie writes that she explored her options and weighed the advantages and disadvantages. Ancker said the reason she chose the Jolie example and what makes it interesting is that it conforms to societal expectations for shared and informed decision making. In this situation the patient gathered relevant information, understood the risks and the options, and engaged in the decision-making process to the extent that she was comfortable.

Ancker noted that there is variability in medical decision making, with some patients choosing to have the doctor take the lead role while other patients would rather be more engaged. Generally, the Jolie example is what is meant by informed decision making in health; informed decision making conducted collaboratively between the patient and a physician is known as shared decision making. Such shared decision making is difficult to achieve in a population with low numeracy skills, especially if the expectation is that patients must really understand risk as part of this shared decision making.

Risk in the medical realm is usually thought of as "epidemiologic risk," which is the probability of developing a certain disease or the number of people who contract a disease over a specific time period over the total number at risk. Many people are also familiar with an economic form of risk, which is the "probability multiplied by utility" concept, Ancker said. As an example, most people in the room would probably agree that a 1 percent risk of developing breast cancer is worse than a 1 percent risk of developing a cold because of the higher "disutility" placed on breast cancer rather than a cold, even when the epidemiologic risks are equivalent. She noted that within the discussion of risk, there is potential for miscommunication with patients if they are thinking about the economic type of risk as opposed to the epidemiologic type of risk.

Uncertainty is also a problem in situations in which it is reasonable to assume there is some risk, but its magnitude is unknown, Ancker said. She noted that a classic example of this is a newly approved drug for which the long-term safety profile is unknown. Another example is confidence intervals where there is a range of plausible estimates for what the risk might be.

Ancker focused her presentation on epidemiologic risks because, she said, in the context of shared decision making the health care professional usually communicates the epidemiologic risks to the patient. At that point the patient is expected to talk about his or her personal utilities, or the personal values the patient holds. This iterative discussion is shared decision making.

According to Ancker, much of the risk communication literature comes from the public health realm in which persuasive communication is the norm and is considered ethically appropriate. In the public health context, informing an individual of his or her personal risk of developing lung cancer is not the goal. The goal is to persuade that individual to quit smoking. This differs from the context of shared decision making, which is a narrower realm. In shared decision making, the goal is to help people have a better understanding of their own risk for a certain disease or condition. As a result, a great deal of the public health risk communication literature focuses on nonquantitative ways of expressing risk, on framing, or on fear appeals and not quantitative risk communication. In shared decision making, however, there is a strong emphasis on ensuring that patients understand their quantitative risk. There is fairly good evidence that people with lower numeracy skills are more reluctant to engage in shared decision making, Ancker said.

Competent use of quantitative information is not solely dependent on the patient's skills, Ancker said. Numeracy is often perceived as a quality, skill, or ability that the patient brings to the situation along with previous knowledge and perception. However, the person providing the information brings a set of skills to the situation as well. This person may be a good communicator or a poor communicator. The competent use of the quantitative information comes from the interaction, not solely from the patient skills. Frequently the discussion is supported or informed by a document, website, or other artifact that contains information. These supports may be designed well or poorly; they may help compensate for low numeracy or increase the numeracy burden on the patient. It is important to remember that the patient is making sense of the information in the context of a social network, a physical environment that may carry risks or no risks, and an information environment that contains news stories and television, radio, and online sources.

Keeping the complexity of the interaction in mind, what are the options for explaining risks? Broadly speaking, information providers can use words, numbers, and pictures. Ancker noted that she would not make a distinction between written and oral or spoken presentation because there has not been sufficient high-quality research about differences between spoken and written communication of numbers.

Evidence indicates that people at the lower levels of numeracy say that they prefer verbal descriptions of risks and that they trust information more when it comes packaged in that format, Ancker said. Words and phrases like "big risk," "small risk," and "common" or "uncommon" are familiar to patients and convey the affective impact that patients say they want. But the disadvantage of this is that such words are not very specific. People also tend to overestimate the number associated with a particular risk word, she said. As a result, it is difficult to use words alone to make good comparisons. For example, "Is a very small risk better or worse than a rare risk?" There is no way to know without more information.

In shared decision making, there is a strong preference for providing information numerically, Ancker said. For example, the International Patient Decision Aid consensus[1] states that patients should be provided with numbers. One option is to present information as percentages. Percentages are generally familiar and are independent of sample size. Two percent of a small group is the same thing as 2 percent of a large group. There can be problems with presenting information in this way, however. Often people do not know how to manipulate percentages and, particularly at lower numeracy levels, do not know how to calculate them. There is good evidence that people perceive them as abstract and may, therefore, feel the information does not apply to them. The difficulty in manipulating percentages is a longstanding problem, Ancker said. She gave the example of providing the risk level and the information that an intervention will reduce that risk by 30 percent. Many times a patient cannot perform the calculation needed to understand what this means for his or her decision making.

Some advocate providing information in terms of frequencies rather than percentages, changing 23 percent to 23 in 100. This is the standard of communication for such factors as genetic risk. Good evidence shows that people perceive this as vivid and personal, said Ancker. Yet this approach has disadvantages. Among the less numerate, this approach may inflate the perceived risk compared to percentages. In addition, there are two other

---

[1] For more information see Elwyn et al. (2006), http://www.ncbi.nlm.nih.gov/pmc/articles/PMC1553508 (accessed October 30, 2013).

problems: denominator neglect and denominator confusion. "Denominator neglect" is the standard term for a longstanding, well-known phenomenon where people, particularly the less numerate, may not recognize that two risks with different denominators are equivalent (e.g., 23 in 100 versus 230 in 1,000) because they focus on the numerators and compare only those two numbers.

"Denominator confusion" is a term coined by Ancker to describe a common misconception that arises when risks are presented to people with different denominators. According to Ancker, there is good evidence that people with lower educational attainment are likely to focus on the numerator and not recognize that 1 in 20,000 is in fact quite a bit smaller than 1 in 5,000. As a result, there has been some promotion of the idea that information should always be presented with the same set of denominators (e.g., a "natural frequencies" format). Presenting the comparison as 4 in 20,000 versus 1 in 20,000 would allow people to make that comparison more easily.

The third option that information providers have is graphics. People like graphics because they are visually interesting and attractive, and they exploit not only learned skills, but also automated visual perception, or things that we do not have to learn. An example is determining which of two bars on a page is larger is an automated task, Ancker said. There is not much, if any, learning involved. As long as the two bars are on the same X-axis or the same horizon, people can automatically tell which one is larger. Judging how much larger one is than the other is also fairly automated. Numeracy skills have something to do with how well an individual can verbalize the size difference, but understanding the differential happens at an automatic level. The learned part is having an understanding of what the two bars mean, knowing the significance of the X axis and Y axis, and how the information applies to the individual. This knowledge is not independent of learned skills at all, Ancker said.

In her review of the graphical literature, Ancker said she identified some core principles that apply to all types of graphics (Ancker and Kaufman, 2007). First, whether the part-to-whole relationship is visible and easily identified is critical to how well people can judge the graphic. Figure 4-1 is an example of a graphic in which the part-to-whole relationship is not visible. The risk represented on the left is 10 percent and on the right, 7 percent. But the graph lacks the context of the entire 100 percent. Extending the Y axis clarifies how the 10 and 7 percent relate to the whole. The graphic on the left inflates the apparent difference and the graphic on the right somewhat minimizes it or at least places it in context. Another example from icon graphics illustrates the point further. Individual risk is a certain number of icons while average risk is another number of icons, but once placed within the context of a larger number, the part-to-whole

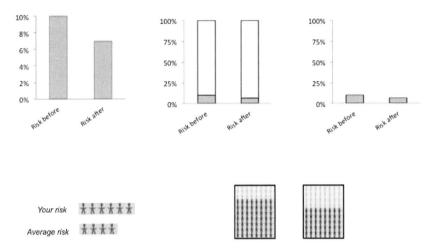

FIGURE 4-1 Judgment is affected by whether the part-to-whole relationship is visible.
SOURCE: Ancker, 2013.

relationship can be shown. The part-to-whole relationship has to be easily visible before people can do this on an automated level, Ancker said.

Figure 4-2 shows two ways of expressing risk where the part-to-whole relationship is visible. Ancker said some good qualitative research suggests that the arrangement on the left does a better job of expressing the idea that anybody can be at risk, that risk is haphazard and random, and that anybody might be affected (Ancker et al., 2011a,b). By contrast, the figure on the right seems more controllable and tidy, as though risk is concen-

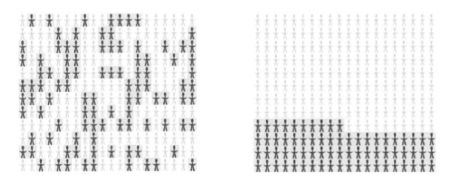

FIGURE 4-2 Graphic representation of risk in a population.
SOURCE: Ancker, 2013.

trated in the population and not distributed throughout. This example shows there are different dimensions of communication effectiveness that must be considered.

The second principle, Ancker said, is that judgments are most accurate when only one dimension varies at a time. In Figure 4-3 there are two bars that change in height and two icon graphics that change in area, height, and width. In general, people are not able to easily judge the difference between two graphics that differ in more than one way. Their perception skills decrease further when circles are used, Ancker added. Pie charts can be a good way of demonstrating part-to-whole relationships, but comparing pie charts of different sizes can lead to confusion.

Ancker noted that three types of graphics have been well studied (see Figure 4-4). Icon graphics, in the form of either smiley faces or small stick figures, are widely used and well understood. There is a very clear visual analogy with the risk information. Icon graphics exploit people's ability to visually process sizes at an automatic level and rely somewhat less on learned information. These graphics are well accepted by people with low numeracy and fulfill the part-to-whole principle requirement.

Bar charts are also fairly well accepted and are familiar to many people,

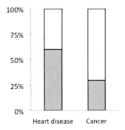

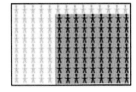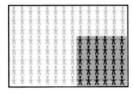

**FIGURE 4-3** Judgments are most accurate when only one dimension varies.
SOURCE: Ancker, 2013.

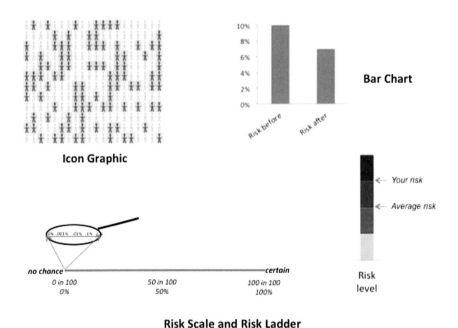

**Risk Scale and Risk Ladder**

FIGURE 4-4 Three common types of graphics.
SOURCE: Ancker, 2013. Horizontal risk scale with magnifier adapted from Woloshin et al., 2000.

Ancker said. She noted that there is some evidence that patients think of them as more abstract and are less able to relate to the information personally when it is in bar chart form. She added that there is also evidence that patients prefer graphics with fewer visual elements in them because the graphics look simpler. Information in a bar graph may seem easier to understand just because there are fewer elements to the graphic.

Finally, risk ladders or risk scales are a type of graphic that is not seen much in health risk communication, but is used more widely in environmental risk communication. The advantage of risk ladders or risk scales is that only one dimension varies at a time, Ancker said. People can easily compare positions along that line. This type of graphic permits the addition of comparative information or some sort of action threshold that indicates that once a risk reaches a certain level, a certain action becomes important or necessary or the risk has exceeded the average for a particular population.

Given that different types of graphics have different advantages and disadvantages, it is important to determine what patients want and find acceptable, Ancker said. Unfortunately, the research has not yielded many clear answers for what patients want. Patients sometimes prefer the more visually simple graphics even if they contain less information. But patients do not necessarily answer comprehension questions better when given information with the graphic type they prefer, and neither do doctors. There is also the question of whether it is better for patients to layer information or have multiple representations of the same information. It is important to guard against the possibility of cognitive overload in the patient instead of better understanding.

Ancker conducted research in which she used an innovative game-like interaction to educate patients about their risk. Instead of merely telling people what their risk was, the game encouraged individuals to click on an icon graphic to uncover which figures in the graphic had the disease. Results showed that the more often people clicked on the icons looking for one with the disease, the more anxious they felt, which was exactly the opposite of what she had hypothesized. The game was attractive and people liked it, but it didn't impart the information in the way that the designers thought it would. She cautioned that this shows that innovative ways of communicating with patients should be studied carefully before they are employed.

Ancker noted that there is another law in addition to the Patient Protection and Affordable Care Act (ACA) of 2010 that is impacting the health care system. The Health Information Technology for Economic and Clinical Health (HITECH) Act of 2009 may not be as obvious to people who are not doctors, but it is changing the practice of medicine. The HITECH Act creates an electronic health record (EHR) incentive program in which doctors and hospitals can receive financial incentives for computerizing their medical records. If they do not make the change, they receive penalties. Over the past 5 years, there has been a massive increase in the number of health care institutions that use EHRs. Many are unaware that there is a mandate that in order to collect the financial incentives, doctors and hospitals must make electronic medical data directly available to patients. Ancker said she believes this is a nationwide experiment in health communication. Patients will be able to access the system and see their medical records, including diagnoses, medication lists, and details of lab tests and radiology reports. There is some concern, however, that this could lead to patient anxiety because they will not understand the meaning of the information they access.

Ancker concluded by listing the areas where she would like to see additional research. The first is the area of novel communication modalities that are available online, such as games and interactive tools. It is not known whether using these types of tools in health and risk communication is beneficial or not. The second area is the experiment in releasing medical records directly to patients, which raises questions such as whether patients will understand the information, how the information will affect shared decision making and risk perception, and what can be done to make this information more useful to patients.

## DISCUSSION

*Moderator: Paul Schyve*

Robert Logan from the National Library of Medicine commented that two important points might get lost in the discussion. First, there is serious research about public health information, the public understanding of science, and news coverage of science and health. A number of journals publish this research, such as the *Journal of Health Communication, Science Communication,* and *Journalism and Mass Communication Quarterly.* Not all of the journals that publish science and health communication research are in PubMed because they also publish a great deal of other social science content that is unrelated to health. Some of content can be accessed easily, but some cannot. Logan said he hopes that PubMed will be able to extend its content to include more of these journals in the future so that health researchers will have better access to this field of study.

The second point, Logan said, is that there are organizations that undertake serious criticism and analysis of health news reporting and how journalists communicate research data to readers. For example, the website Holloway mentioned in her talk, HealthNewsReview.org, offers critiques of the reporting from major news organizations on a daily basis. Logan also commented that the Association of Health Care Journalists engages in a great deal of professional development in the field and encouraged those present to visit the Association's website, healthjournalism.org. He added that the *Columbia Journalism Review* also has excellent criticism of how the news media covers health insurance–related issues.

Rima Rudd, roundtable member, noted that the presentations confirmed the notion that journalism is public health's best partner and that training journalists in how to communicate science and health concepts is vital. Rudd said that mathematical terms are often taken for granted and that more attention should be paid to explaining terms such as "normal," "range," and "risk." She noted that individuals and cultures react differently to the word "risk" and related an anecdote from a colleague that in certain Native American cultures, risk was assumed to convey inevitability. Efforts should not just be about communicating numbers, Rudd said, but also concepts. Rudd also recommended a tool developed by Mosenthal and Kirsch (1998) called the PMOSE-IKirsch assessment tool that rates the complexity of documents and document elements, including charts and graphs.[2] Ancker replied that the PMOSE-IKirsch tool is a great resource. She added that every component of health communication, including the clinician, the patient, and the document or materials used, should be included in determining ways to make communication better because miscommunication arises from a problem in the interaction between parties, not just from a patient's inability to understand. Rudd noted that the idea of health literacy arising from interactions rather than being embedded in an individual is a central point of the Institute of Medicine's 2004 report on health literacy.[3]

Patrick McGarry, roundtable member, asked whether any studies had been done on people's perceptions of case studies versus population-based statistics. He noted that although suicide is low prevalence, it is a very real problem. Journalists must be careful how they present the data and what conclusions they draw for their readers. Holloway answered that she was unaware of any research that looks specifically at case studies versus population studies and its impact on media coverage. There is always a tension in journalism between focusing on personal stories versus population-level data. Holloway said that when a journalist can take a personal story and relate it to the larger population, it has more effect, but that journalists must be careful because sometimes using people's personal stories can feel exploitive to readers.

Susan Pisano, another roundtable member, commented that medical journals assume that their audience consists only of practicing physicians, yet members of the public are reading these journals more and more often. No effort is made to translate these studies into something that would be easier for journalists to write about or for the average person to understand. Holloway responded that some medical journals think about the members of their audience that are not physicians. They provide video clips, press releases, and other information. Sometimes these help journalists to report more accurately, but they can also be misleading and manipulative. Journalists should be careful about relying too much on a single source that may be advancing a particular interest. The time demands on journalists can lead to them relying too much on press releases rather than doing their own reporting. They need to be careful about that, she said.

Ruth Parker, roundtable member, pointed out that the field of health literacy is somewhat nascent, and that she believes health literacy is entering its second generation. This has offered a chance for reflection in the field and an opportunity to chart the course for the next 20 years. Parker

---

[2] The tool can be found online at http://www.hsph.harvard.edu/healthliteracy/files/2012/09/pmose.pdf (accessed November 3, 2013).

[3] The report *Health Literacy: A Prescription to End Confusion* can be found online at http://www.nap.edu/catalog.php?record_id=10883 (accessed November 5, 2013).

said that health communicators and people in the media are natural allies and asked if the speakers had any thoughts or suggestions on how to forge stronger ties between the two fields. Ancker answered that in some ways, health communicators and journalists are not natural allies. For example, journalists do not focus on literacy differences within their readership. Journalists tend to assume that their readers are all at the same level, she said. Journalists are interested in getting information to the public, but do not see any additional level of explanation or translation as being within their role. In addition, Ancker said, journalists are often skeptical about their sources even when those sources are doctors or public health authorities. To do a good job, journalists have to stand a little apart and avoid the risk of being seen as a spokesperson for a particular view. Ancker said she would encourage more communication between the two fields, but that their perspectives are very different. Holloway agreed and added there is some opportunity to work with professional associations and strengthen training in health communication for journalists.

As a follow-up, Parker gave the example of the upcoming enrollment period for the health care insurance marketplaces opening under the ACA. She noted that there are people who are interested in communicating to the public about how to use the exchanges in ways that are understandable and actionable. Journalists are also interested in providing accurate information to the public. Parker asked how the two groups could work together to provide accurate and usable information. Holloway answered that in that example, the best way forward would be for the health communicators to contact individual journalists and publications. But she cautioned that the journalists would not see it as a collaboration, but rather information provided to them so they could report on it independently.

Paul Schyve, roundtable member, commented that in Chicago public officials have turned to investigative reporters to advise them on oversight issues. The reasoning behind this is that reporters are trained to be skeptical and determine the validity of information for themselves rather than relying on the assurances of others. Schyve added that reporters and health communicators could learn from each other without necessarily collaborating on work.

Cindy Brach, another roundtable member, said she was interested in Ancker's point that people do not necessarily better understand the graphics they prefer. The research on this topic is mixed. Generally people prefer simpler materials, but there is not strong evidence that this improves comprehension. She asked if any research shows that presenting information a certain way will improve comprehension. Ancker answered that there is a concept within informatics called "task technology fit," which is that in human factors in informatics, there is no single technology that solves all problems. A technology's usefulness is dependent on the context of the task.

She added that the research literature on graphics is confounded by the fact that different people are asking subjects to do different tasks, and thus getting different results. For example, if a researcher asks people to compare icon graphs to bar charts, but only one of the graphs for comparison makes the part-to-whole relationship visible, then the research results are unreliable. In addition, there is another layer of variability, which is that familiarity has an effect on comprehension. This means there is a sociological element to understanding graphics because some types of graphics will be familiar to different audiences at different times. Researchers are making inferences based on studies about how people are going to relate to electronic information, but that relationship will change over time.

Roundtable member Steven Rush asked about the effectiveness of "infographics" for presenting information visually in the news or for providing health information and reminders. Ancker answered that there is a growing emphasis on visual communication and that, in many ways, this is an improvement over previous methods. The effectiveness of a specific type of communication or piece of information would depend on the context both in terms of the communication itself and the audience. Rush then asked if there is a way to calculate the numeracy burden of a specific piece of information or material. Ancker said she is not aware of a way to measure the demands of a document or education material, but she would be interested in developing one and in shifting the focus away from measuring the skills of the patient. Rudd added that doctoral students in her program had adapted Apter's hierarchy for numerical information by adding numbers to produce a scale that helps determine the numeric burden of information. This method is in its early stages and has not been tested, but it is a first step toward developing a tool that measures numeracy burden. Holloway added that within journalism, there is a growing emphasis on data visualization, and a great deal of work is being done on how to best present various types of information so they are easily understood by the reader.

Benard Dreyer, roundtable member, asked the presenters about the best way to communicate risk and risk reduction to patients. Ancker answered that showing the part-to-whole relationship is an important part of communicating risk and risk reduction because it gives people context. She also noted that providers might have different goals for the communication depending on the situation, and that this would affect how information was presented. For example, a clinician who is trying to get a patient to quit smoking would present information differently than one who was trying to help a patient choose between two therapeutic options. Dreyer commented that a good example of the difficulty of risk communication is vaccines. Because most of the diseases that are vaccinated against have been all but eradicated, the absolute risk reduction from immunizations is quite small. The relative risk reduction, however, is very high. Dreyer said that if he focuses on absolute risk reduction, then vaccination might not seem worth it. Yet if people do not take the vaccines, these diseases could reappear. Ancker replied that there are a number of issues contained in that example. This might be an area in which non-quantitative risk communication is more effective. Quantitative risk communication is not the only tool available and is not always the most appropriate tool.

Schyve pointed out that this discussion is another example of the ethical ramifications of many of these issues. The ethics of a specific situation and the goals must be considered. George Isham, roundtable chair, asked whether it would be ethical for a professional in a situation where the vast number of patients cannot evaluate the information to consciously present information in a way calculated to persuade rather than inform. He reminded the group of the controversy surrounding the change in the recommendations regarding mammograms. In that case the change in absolute risk was very small, but many women feel that risk on a personal level. Isham concluded that there are serious ethical issues around the topic of numeracy and health literacy and the responsibility of professionals to communicate ethically, and that those issues should be explored. Ancker agreed that there are ethical issues involved in whether a health communicator's job is to persuade or merely give information. She stressed that the issue is highly context specific. For example, society and the public health community are very comfortable with using scare appeals to persuade people to quit smoking. Both would feel differently about attempting to persuade people to get more X-rays or take more prescription drugs. She noted that professional communities will nearly always have more information than the general public and that they will always have some control over how that information is communicated.

Schyve ended the discussion by noting that these ethical issues will require a great deal more discussion and analysis in the future.

## REFERENCES

Ancker, J. 2013. *Issues and challenges in the era of shared decision making: Explaining risk and uncertainty*. PowerPoint presentation, Institute of Medicine Workshop on Health Literacy and Numeracy, Washington, DC, July 18.

Ancker, J. S., and D. Kaufman. 2007. Rethinking health numeracy: A multidisciplinary literature review. *Journal of the American Medical Informatics Association* 14(6):713-721.

Ancker, J. S., E. U. Weber, and R. Kukafka. 2011a. Effects of game-like interactive graphics on risk perceptions and decisions. *Medical Decision Making* 31:130.

Ancker, J. S., E. U. Weber, and R. Kukafka. 2011b. Effects of arrangement of stick figures on estimate of proportion in risk graphics. *Medical Decision Making* 31:143.

Elwyn, G., A. O'Connor, D. Stacey, R. Volk, A. Edwards, A. Coulter, R. Thomson, A. Barratt, M. Barry, S. Bernstein, P. Butow, A. Clarke, V. Entwistle, D. Feldman-Stewart, M. Holmes-Rovner, H. Llewellyn-Thomas, N. Moumjid, A. Mulley, C. Ruland, K. Sepucha, A. Sykes, T. Whelan, and The International Patient Decision Aids Standards (IPDAS) Collaboration. 2006. Developing a quality criteria framework for patient decision aids: Online international Delphi Consensus process. *British Medical Journal* 333(7565):417.

Gould, S. J. 1985. The median isn't the message. *Discover*, June.

Maier, S. R. 2012. Numbers in the news: A mathematics audit of a daily newspaper. *Journalism Studies* 3(4):507-519.

Mosenthal, P., and I. Kirsch. 1998. A new measure for assessing document complexity: The PMOSE/IKirsch document readability formula. *Journal of Adolescent and Adult Literacy* 41:638-657.

Raeburn, P. 2013. Shaky ground: Speculating on the causes of suicide. *Knight Science Journalism Tracker*, May 6.

Schwitzer, G. 2008. How do U.S. journalists cover treatments, tests, products, and procedures?: An evaluation of 500 stories. *PLoS Medicine* 5(5):e95.

Twenge, J. 2013. How long can you wait to have a baby? *The Atlantic*, July/August.

Voss, M. 2002. Checking the pulse: Midwestern reporters' opinions on their ability to report health care news. *American Journal of Public Health* 92(7):1158-1160.

Woloshin, S., L. M. Schwartz, S. Byram, B. Fischhoff, and H. G. Welch. 2000. A new scale for assessing perceptions of chance: A validation study. *Medical Decision Making* 20(3):298-307.

# 5

# Strategies for Effective Communication

The final panel addressed several strategies for effectively communicating numeracy concepts. The presenters were Robert Krughoff from Consumers' CHECKBOOK, an independent, nonprofit consumer information organization; Brian Zikmund-Fisher from the Department of Health Behavior and Health Education at the University of Michigan School of Public Health; and Michael Wolf from the Health Literacy and Learning Program within the Feinberg School of Medicine at Northwestern University.

## EXAMPLES OF EFFECTIVE DISPLAY OF HEALTH PLAN INFORMATION

*Robert Krughoff, J.D.*
*President,*
*Consumers' CHECKBOOK*

Krughoff said his presentation would give details of one practical solution to help consumers choose the right health plan for them. Consumers' CHECKBOOK has a health plan comparison tool that can be adapted by the health insurance marketplaces opened under the Patient Protection and Affordable Care Act (ACA). This tool can simplify the process of choosing a health insurance policy for consumers so that their choices are easier and also the right choices for that consumer. The purpose of the tool is to help consumers with little knowledge of insurance or the health care system without requiring much time or training. The context for Consumers' CHECKBOOK's recommendations is the nonprofit organization's decades of experience producing websites and publications rating a variety of consumer products, from hospitals to auto insurers. No Consumers' CHECKBOOK website or publication carries any advertising; the organization's products are supported by consumers who pay to access the information. Krughoff said this provides motivation for the organization to produce information the people find valuable and useful. Krughoff said the most relevant aspect of Consumers' CHECKBOOK experience is that for 34 years they have produced CHECKBOOK's Guide to Health Plans for Federal Employees.[1]

Certain features are considered key for a health plan comparison tool, Krughoff said. First, a single dollar amount actuarial estimate of average total cost, including premium and out-of-pocket cost estimates for people with similar characteristics to the consumer, must be provided. A good comparison tool will also include the user's range of risk for each plan, giving the total cost for good years and bad years and the probability of the consumer having those types of years. There should be an all-plan provider directory that lets the user see immediately which doctors are approved by the plan, Krughoff explained. Finally, it should include a summary rating for each plan's care and service quality that the user can personalize based on the things that are a priority to that user.

According to Krughoff, consumers tend to be most interested in cost comparisons. The most common cost comparison tool for consumers who have a choice in health plans is the benefits description model. This model shows the consumer the benefits and coverage details, such as deductibles, copayments, and out-of-pocket limits associated with each plan. The weakness of this model, Krughoff said, is that research has shown that many consumers do not understand the terms and are not able to do the calculations required to understand this information. Yet even those with very high numeracy skills have trouble making good choices given this information because they do not know the likelihood that they will need different types of health services and the fees for those services.

Other models have been developed in an effort to simplify the cost comparison process, Krughoff said. He explained that one solution is the known-usage model, which compares plans by having the consumer estimate the number of provider visits and prescriptions that will be required in the next year. The model then gives an estimate of the cost of these services. This is time consuming to do for each family member, Krughoff said. But

---

[1] More information can be found at http://www.checkbook.org/newhig2/hig.cfm (accessed October 30, 2013).

the main problem with this approach is that it does not account for the risk of an unforeseen health event that may be very expensive.

Another model that simplifies health insurance choice is the Enroll UX2014 website that was funded and developed by a number of foundations.[2] One feature of that model is that it asks the consumer's preferences up front and then filters plan choices based on those preferences. For example, the model will ask if a deductible above a certain amount is acceptable, if a consumer will consider a health maintenance organization (HMO), or if a specific doctor must be available through the plan. The choices presented to the consumer are based on the answers to those questions. Krughoff said the weakness of this model is that it eliminates choices before the consumer even sees them. Consumers do not realize they may be giving up thousands of dollars by answering questions a certain way. Krughoff said consumers can make false assumptions, such as that a low deductible is the best way to save money or a low premium is a sure way to save money. This is often not the case.

Plan standardization is another method of simplification. Krughoff said there is merit to this approach because it allows consumers to compare premiums within a specific benefit package. The problem is that it is important to compare across packages as well because individuals have vastly different needs, and a package that might save one consumer a lot of money might prove to be very expensive for another consumer. In addition, limiting the packages reduces flexibility in developing benefit designs for consumers.

The Consumers' CHECKBOOK model uses data from the Medical Expenditure Panel Survey and other sources to estimate the likelihood of various levels of usage and the charges related to that level of usage. From this, the model estimates a single dollar amount that is combined with the premium to give consumers one number that they can use to compare plans, Krughoff said. In addition to average costs, the tool offers people the option of seeing what the costs would be in a very good year and in a very bad year. In recent years, Krughoff said, the Medicare Plan Finder has adopted the same approach.

Krughoff said it is very challenging to design a quality comparison tool that does not require strong literacy or numeracy skills. One challenge is that consumers do not attribute differences in health results to differences in plan quality. They tend to attribute differences in health results to the providers the consumer chooses within the plan or to the consumer's individual behavior. If patients are going to be involved and engaged in thinking about plan quality, they need to be educated on how plans can impact quality. Another challenge is that it may be hard for consumers to interpret differences in plan scores. To simplify presentation, Consumers'

---

[2] More information can be found at http://www.ux2014.org (accessed November 1, 2013).

CHECKBOOK uses a five-star rating system, but that does not give a sense of scale to the consumer. Two plans might have big differences in some categories, but still end up in the same quintile, or small differences, and end up in different quintiles. Attempting to get beyond this simplistic rating system, however, requires a level of complexity that is difficult for people to manage. Krughoff said that consumers want, and Consumers' CHECKBOOK provides, a summary measure of plan quality. In addition, Consumers' CHECKBOOK gives them the opportunity to get more detail about the summary measure and to give their own personalized weights to various dimensions of quality and thus create a personalized overall quality score. The challenge with quality measures and with other elements of comparison tools is that if consumers are forced into too much detail, they become disengaged.

Krughoff gave a tour of the tool that Consumers' CHECKBOOK has developed to overcome these challenges. The tool is based on the website used by federal employees to choose plans from the Federal Employees Health Benefits Program and adjusted for use with the health insurance exchanges. Krughoff said that Consumers' CHECKBOOK has learned that people receive information better in some formats than in others. As a result their websites provide information in text, audio, and video formats.

Personal and family information is imported into the tool from the eligibility module of an exchange, so a consumer does not have to enter that information twice. The first step of the comparison tool is to answer questions on self-reported health status. According to Krughoff, the Medicare Expenditure Panel Survey asks about self-reported health status, which is a very good predictor of usage. Next, the consumer can identify some medical procedures or expenditures that are expected within the next year, such as childbirth or a hip replacement. The consumer can also enter the names of one or more doctors that he or she would like to have available through the plan, and the tool then automatically shows them which of these providers are in each plan. This step comes with a warning to consumers that if certain providers are really important, they should check with those providers to make sure the plan will include them the following year.

The results are presented in a way that highlights average yearly costs, which is a combination of the yearly premium minus any tax subsidy and the costs that the consumer may pay out of pocket. Krughoff said the tool also provides consumers with the most that they would pay in a very high-usage year under each plan. This is important because the information given by individual plans may not be presented in a straightforward manner or may lack some information, such as failing to include drug costs in the out-of-pocket maximum. The quality measures are presented simply using the five-star rating method, but consumers are able to personalize the components included in the quality score. According to Krughoff, more than

60 percent of people make their plan choice based on the summary page, which includes total annual cost, highest possible cost, quality measures, and whether the consumer's preferred doctors are in the plan. Consumers' CHECKBOOK surveys and user testing have indicated that this is the information consumers want and the way they want it to be presented, he said.

More detailed information is available for those who want it, Krughoff said. Smaller numbers of plans can be compared side by side in more detail, for example. The consumer can also see more detailed cost information, including comparing a low-cost year and a high-cost year and the probability of one of those years occurring. Consumers can also look for plans with coverage for certain services, such as fertility treatments or acupuncture. They can also find out what the members of each plan have to say about various quality measures. This is helpful for those who are interested in a certain aspect of a plan's quality rating, such as customer service or availability of doctors, and of others' experiences in those areas.

Consumers also have the option of eliminating broad categories of plans that they do not want, such as HMOs or high-deductible plans, Krughoff said. But this option is offered after all of the plans have been presented to the user in the summary page. This way the consumer is less likely to exclude plans that would be a good fit without even knowing it.

Krughoff noted that it is possible to give consumers the information they need while keeping the format simple and understandable and allowing them to decide the level of personalization and detail.

### WHY ARE YOU GIVING ME THIS NUMBER?: COMMUNICATING QUANTITATIVE INFORMATION FOR DECISION MAKING

*Brian J. Zikmund-Fisher, Ph.D.*
*Department of Health Behavior and Health Education,*
*University of Michigan*

Zikmund-Fisher said his presentation was not a review of the evidence on numeracy, but an argument that he hoped would be provocative. He began with the example of a fictional person called "Robert" (Zikmund-Fisher, 2013a). Robert is a stereotypical middle-age man living in the United States. He is not as healthy as he should be or wishes to be because he has hypertension, is overweight, and does not get enough exercise. Robert decides to use an online risk calculator to find out whether he is at risk for cardiovascular disease. The risk calculator asks Robert his blood pressure, his weight and height, his cholesterol, and a few other pieces of information before providing the result. Robert learns that his 10-year risk of cardiovascular disease is 14.52 percent. But Robert is confused; he still does not know whether he is at high risk or not.

The number provided to Robert—14.52 percent—may be the best estimate of his risk of disease that modern medicine could give him, Zikmund-Fisher said. Yet that number does not meet Robert's need for information. Robert's risk is not being effectively communicated to him through that number. Zikmund-Fisher said there are several problems with the way that his risk of cardiovascular disease was communicated to Robert. First, there is the level of precision. Although it is common for risk calculators to give numeric risk estimates to two decimal points, it is not necessary or beneficial. Research has shown that an integer is considered more believable as well as easier to remember than a more precise representation of risk (Witteman et al., 2011).

More important, Zikmund-Fisher added, is the fact that Robert did not get the information that he needed from the number. Robert needed to know whether he was at high risk of developing cardiovascular disease or not. Merely giving him a number does not answer that question for him. Decision-making research uses the term "information evaluability" (Hsee, 1996), which means that the meaning of a number depends on its context and whether the number can be evaluated by itself or requires reference standards to convey meaning.

For example, Zikmund-Fisher said, if workshop participants were shown a number that corresponds to the level of dioxin in blood, many would not know how to evaluate that data (i.e., to know whether it represents a high or low concentration or even whether being high or low is good or bad). The sense of confusion that workshop participants likely felt when presented with information about dioxin is the same feeling that many patients have when they are given any type of number in a health or medical situation without the contextual knowledge to explain whether the number is good or bad. Another example might be a person with type 2 diabetes who is working to improve glycemic control. If this person starts with a hemoglobin A1c measurement of 9.3 percent and after some time lowers that number to 8.3 percent, there is an important question: Will that person know whether the difference between those two numbers is large or small? Experts know that hemoglobin A1c values exist in a relatively narrow range, and thus a change of 1 percent is important. However, if the person with diabetes does not know that fact, then his or her ability to make sense of their test data is limited. Zikmund-Fisher said health professionals are trained to have the contextual knowledge for the numbers they give to patients, but they may forget that the patients often do not have the same background and hence will have a hard time deriving meaning from numeric information.

An example of information being presented with some contextual information is the National Cancer Institute's breast cancer risk assessment tool, Zikmund-Fisher said. The tool presents an individual's risk compared to the average woman's risk.[3] A woman whose results show that she is above average may not remember her numerical risk, but she will likely note that she is in more danger of developing breast cancer than the average woman. Whether she will understand her risk in absolute terms is difficult to determine.

Information evaluability is linked to decision making, Zikmund-Fisher said. Easy-to-evaluate data have intrinsic meaning. For example, when speaking about health insurance plans and cost, an individual knows how much $100 is worth to him or her. People also know the difference between two doctors who are 10 minutes away versus an hour away. They do not need a reference standard to evaluate those numbers. They might, however, need a reference standard to make sense of an unfamiliar laboratory value or a breast cancer risk statistic. Decision-making research has found that hard-to-evaluate data given without a reference standard are generally ignored. It is possible to distort people's perceptions by choosing one reference standard over another, but in the absence of any reference standard, the information receives no attention at all.

Zikmund-Fisher drew the analogy that information evaluability is related to numeracy in the way that functional health literacy is related to health literacy. It is the key to enabling someone to function in the numerical world—not just to recognize the number, but also to draw the meaning they need from the number to make the choices they need to make.

Zikmund-Fisher showed an example of a table from an electronic health record (EHR) (see Figure 5-1) that gave a patient's lab results along with the normal range for those types of laboratory tests. He noted that patients are being exposed to information presented in this way more often because of EHRs and patient portals. The numeracy-related task for patients with information of this type is to recognize whether the values of their tests are outside of the range of normal. Some patients will be able to do that and others will not, Zikmund-Fisher said.

Yet, a better question to ask, said Zikmund-Fisher, is: Is this the information that is most important to the patient? Perhaps it is more important for patients to understand harm anchors or thresholds for action than the normal range. Using a different reference standard can give the patient information that is clearer and actionable. It is important to think about structuring information in ways that empower the patient, Zikmund-Fisher said.

Zikmund-Fisher said another problem with Robert's story is that he

---

[3] The tool is available at http://www.cancer.gov/bcrisktool/Default.aspx (accessed November 1, 2013).

**Component Results**

| Component | Your Value | Standard Range | Units |
|---|---|---|---|
| WBC Count | 5.2 | 4.0 - 10.0 | K/MM3 |
| Hemoglobin | 15.8 | 13.5 - 17.0 | g/dl |
| Hematocrit | 44.7 | 40.0 - 50.0 | % |
| Platelet Count | 145 | 150 - 400 | K/MM3 |
| RBC Count | 4.71 | 4.40 - 5.70 | M/MM3 |
| Mean Corpuscular Volume | 94.9 | 79.0 - 99.0 | fl |
| Mean Corpuscular Hgb | 33.5 | 27.0 - 32.0 | pg |
| Mean Corpuscular Hgb Conc. | 35.3 | 32.0 - 35.0 | G/DL |
| Red Cell Distribution Width | 11.7 | 11.5 - 15.0 | % |
| Mean Platelet Volume | 11.1 | 9.0 - 12.2 | fl |

FIGURE 5-1 Can patients *use* this? An example of information from an electronic health record.
SOURCE: Zikmund-Fisher, 2013b.

was only given a number without any way of visualizing his cardiovascular risk. Zikmund-Fisher noted that he has done a number of studies that support the use of icon arrays as a way to communicate health information visually. One problem with these arrays, however, is that they are not easy to create with standard software packages. A tool, available at iconarray.com, has been developed at the University of Michigan that enables people to make and download icon displays in an effort to promote communication using more effective graphics.

Given that visual displays of information are often effective ways to communicate information, Zikmund-Fisher asked if Robert even needed a number. In areas outside of health, such as investing and financial management or consumer products, data are often presented qualitatively to facilitate decision making. For example, investment websites break risk down into categories. The potential investor can see which investments are high risk and high return versus low risk and low return without seeing any numbers. Consumer product reliability data are also often not reported in numeric form. They are reported in icon form because that best helps consumers understand the trade-offs involved in choosing one product over another. Zikmund-Fisher stressed that he believes data are important. However, conscious choices can be made to focus less on detail and more on the overall goal of the communication. Health may also be an area where a similar trade-off is appropriate. Patients have varying data needs, he said, and all communications are not equally informative.

Zikmund-Fisher noted that risk information exists on a spectrum (Zikmund-Fisher, 2013a). A risk communication designed to communicate all possible risks can be very simple, whereas a risk communication designed to quantify incremental risk reduction associated with a particular therapy may be more complex. Considering the example of Robert again, Robert is looking for motivation to act. He wants a categorical communication that aligns with that goal, which he did not get from the risk calculator. Zikmund-Fisher said that communicators must always consider the congruence of the data types and formats given to patients to their immediate and specific needs. In other words, give people the right tool at the right time.

Patients have many needs with regard to information and communication that must be met to allow them to navigate the health care system and make the best choices for their situation. Zikmund-Fisher said this often leads health providers and communicators to feel the need to tell patients every piece of information known about their diagnosis or situation. Research shows, however, that this is not always what is best for the patients. The recipient of the message can be so overwhelmed by the data and the tasks involved in interpreting it that the information is lost. Zikmund-Fisher gave as an example an animation tool that he and some colleagues had developed to communicate information and aid in decision making (Zikmund-Fisher et al., 2011). The people using the tool became so involved in learning how to manipulate it that they lost sight of the information it was intended to convey. The lesson here is to focus on what people need to know and then give them that alone.

If the goal of the communication is for the person to assess whether they are at high risk or low risk, does that need a number? If the goal is for a person to make a careful trade-off between two courses of action, then a number may be necessary. Zikmund-Fisher stressed that he was not advocating withholding information, but rather recognizing that there is a difference between what needs to be seen initially and what needs to be seen eventually. Seeing information for the first time and trying to make sense of it is a different task than when the information has been absorbed. Communications need to be designed with goals and tasks involved in the communications in mind, he concluded.

## EFFECTIVELY COMMUNICATING MEDICATION INSTRUCTIONS

*Michael Wolf, Ph.D., M.P.H.*
*Health Literacy and Learning Program,*
*Feinberg School of Medicine, Northwestern University*

Wolf said he was invited to talk about effectively communicating medication instructions, and he would narrow the topic to the numeracy and problem-solving skills required in medication use. Medication is one of the most common tools in medicine to promote health and control chronic disease, but using this tool is difficult and challenging for people.

First, Wolf said, it is necessary to deconstruct the task and ask, "Why is taking medicine so hard?" Medication use is a dynamic task, with medications often being added and taken away from a patient's regimen as well as dosages being increased and decreased (see Box 5-1). There are multidrug regimens with variable doses. Although the tendency is to think of medications as always occurring in pill form, in reality there are multiple devices to deliver medications. Medicines are prescribed in tapered and escalating, daily and nondaily, and as-needed or extended dosages. In addition, some patients must handle medications from multiple prescribers and pharmacies, increasing the complexity. Insurance can also have an effect on medication. As coverage changes, medication can change from brand name to generic, changing the appearance of the medication. It can also be difficult to synchronize refills, which can lead to multiple trips to the pharmacy.

Chronic conditions are on the rise, said Wolf, and patients are taking more and more medications. The focus must be on regimen use, safety, and adherence. The skill set required to manage medication tasks includes not only numeracy but other skills, such as reading, attention, and problem solving. All of these skills are related, Wolf said. Research based on data from the National Institute on Aging has shown there is a strong correlation between literacy and numeracy. High reading skills are strongly associated with being able to perform health tasks, and numeracy skills are associated

---

**BOX 5-1**
**Why Is It So Hard to Take Medication?**

- A dynamic behavior (*adding, changing, removing medication*)
- Multidrug regimens, variable doses
- Multiple devices (*pill, injection, inhaler, liquid, nasal, eye drops, lotions, etc.*)
- Tapered and escalating doses
- Doses dependent on measurement (*i.e., weight, blood sugar*)
- Daily versus non-daily medicines
- Limited-duration versus chronic, extended-duration medicines
- "PRN" (Pro Re Nata) or "as needed" and seasonal medicines
- Multiple prescribers, multiple pharmacies, variable instructions
- Brand versus generic drugs (*variable trade dress*)
- Unsynchronized fill dates from pharmacy

SOURCE: Wolf, 2013.

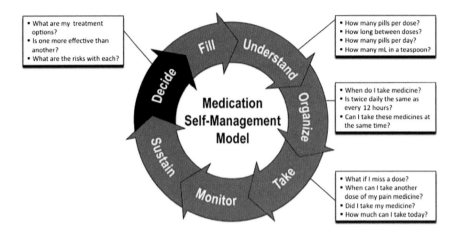

FIGURE 5-2 Deconstruct the task: A medication self-management model.
SOURCE: Wolf, 2013.

with the ability to perform tasks around medication use. But the combination of reading and numeracy skills is far more significant than either of them alone because medication use requires such a diverse set of skills.

Wolf proposed a model that he is developing with a colleague as a way of further deconstructing the task of taking medications and understanding targets for intervention (see Figure 5-2). First, there is the decision point for which medication and how to take it. Questions concerning options, effectiveness, and risk must be answered. Next there are questions about dosage and timing that must be addressed by the provider and patient. There are further questions regarding how to handle unusual situations or a break in the routine. People have a difficult time getting answers to these questions because providers have not adequately communicated with them regarding the medications, Wolf said.

A great deal of research shows that people have trouble taking their medications, Wolf said. Half of people misunderstand common dosing instructions (Davis et al., 2006). Patients' abilities to decipher the instruction "Take two pills by mouth twice daily" depended on their literacy levels. The instructions could be written more clearly, however, to make them easier for everyone to understand. The National Assessment of Adult Literacy found that 60 percent of patients struggle with auxiliary instructions for medication dosage. A study done at New York University found that one in four make large dosing errors with pediatric liquid medication (Yin et al., 2008). Eighty-five percent of patients may unnecessarily overcomplicate drug regimens. Providers may not help people understand the most efficient way to take their medicines or work with them to integrate the dosing instructions of different medications. Regimen complexity, along with cost, is one of the most common reasons that people stop taking medications, Wolf said.

For over-the-counter (OTC) pain medications, one in four may exceed maximum daily dosages. Wolf cited research he conducted that showed that consumers often combined products when they should not have and commonly exceeded the maximum daily dose limit. Many retail stores have large OTC pain medication sections with a wide variety of products, Wolf said. Consumers are very familiar with these products, often having used them for decades. How many people are reading the bottles for new information or new warnings? There are many differences between products, and consumers may not be paying attention to how those differences should affect dosing.

The consequences of this complexity are that half of adults demonstrate inadequate adherence to prescription regimens. Such a low level of adherence is commonly found in the cardiovascular and diabetes research. Wolf said that only adherence to HIV medications is consistently higher, but that is because adherence to HIV medication has been a main focus for researchers and providers. According to Wolf, 20 percent of new prescriptions are abandoned and never filled at the pharmacy and more than 1.5 million adverse drug reactions occur annually, with a quarter million of those occurring in children. He also noted that one-half of acute liver failure cases in the United States are caused by acetaminophen overdose. Sixty-one percent of these cases are unintentional, and exceeding the maximum dose was identified as the root cause, Wolf said.

The task of taking medication is complicated and the consequences are significant, Wolf said. This is a multifaceted problem that requires a multifaceted solution. First, medication labeling can be standardized and improved. A great deal of work is being done in this area, Wolf said, especially in California and by the U.S. Pharmacopeia. Second is to increase the prevalence and quality of patient counseling. Improving drug labeling is an important task, but it is not the only thing that will help simplify medication use. More provider–patient communication is needed, Wolf said, to help people understand these complex tasks and they need to stay connected with patients because the task is always changing. Finally, a variety of support tools needs to be engineered for different contexts. These interventions could help people perform the numeracy tasks required and check to make sure that the correct information is heard and understood by patients. This can help simplify the behavior that patients have to perform on a daily basis and prevent it from becoming obtrusive in their lives.

An example of a useful tool is the universal medication schedule, Wolf said (see Figure 5-3). A great deal of evidence establishes the universal medi-

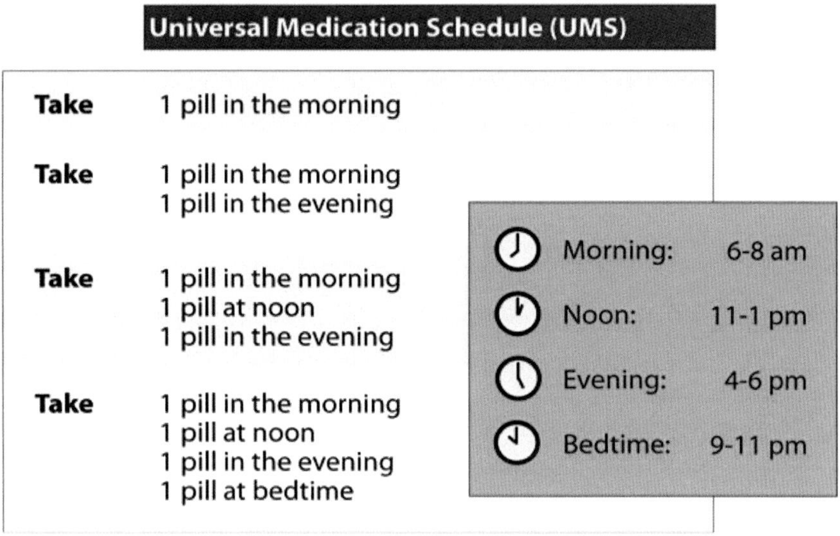

**FIGURE 5-3** Universal medication schedule.
SOURCE: Wolf, 2013.

cation schedule as a best practice, and Wolf said he believes making it standard, and incorporating it into EHRs and pharmacy labels, would lead to better patient understanding of medication instructions. Imagine how much clearer it would be if all medication labels read morning, noon, evening, or bedtime instead of "once every 12 hours" or "twice daily," Wolf said.

Wolf is also working to develop a tool that can be used at the point of prescribing, not just for one medicine but for an entire regimen. This tool would use the universal medication schedule for the entire regimen. Eventually the tool could be put onto a patient portal so that patients can receive updated information about their regimens without waiting for a new appointment or for instructions to be mailed. Working with the new medium of the EHR brings new opportunities to meet patient needs. There is also important work being done at New York University on improving communication about medications, Wolf said. Their research has shown that using icons when dosing with syringes and cups can have a powerful effect on patient understanding. Another tool that is under development is a standardized prescription drug facts box on the medication label. The information attempts to both quantify and qualify risks. This tool, however, is still being refined because some patients have found it confusing.

Other efforts have focused on improving medication guides, building bridges between providers and pharmacists, and increasing the prevalence of counseling, Wolf said. There is also a large body of research around a very complicated medication context, congestive heart failure, which addresses issues such as how to communicate with a patient when medication use is dependent on other factors such as weight. Wolf said there are also a number of external aids that have been less tested, but show some promise, such as blister packs or mobile phone apps that help with medication management. He concluded by saying that there is a lot of ongoing work in this field and best practices are continuing to develop.

## DISCUSSION

### Moderator: Paul Schyve

Benard Dreyer, roundtable member, commented on the importance of connecting the pharmacist and physician to better manage medication use for patients. He asked how it might be possible to better integrate pharmacists into the process. Wolf answered that there have been a few studies on embedding pharmacists into primary care practices, but that for most practices this would not be cost effective. Adding pharmacists as part of a medical home is another idea that is currently being explored, but it is not certain whether this could be a sustainable model. There are also several demonstration projects being undertaken with some national pharmacy chains that explore ways to leverage technology to provide direct support to patients by linking and partnering with other providers, Wolf said. There is a question, however, of whether medical practices can give a pharmacist who is not an employee access to a patient's EHR to use that information to provide medication reviews and decision support. Wolf added that he thought that things would change when there is reimbursement for medication therapy management for those 65 and older or with complex chronic conditions.

Darren DeWalt, roundtable member, asked whether the 14 percent risk of cardiovascular disease mentioned in Zikmund-Fisher's presentation would be considered high. He said that, as a clinician, he would consider it a high risk, but that another clinician might not. Zikmund-Fisher commented that this question got to the point of the presentation. One cannot say from the number whether a person should be taking a particular set of actions, but this brings back the original question of whether this risk calculator is of value. If the purpose of the risk calculator is to serve as a signal to action, the 14 percent estimate does not fulfill that purpose because it is not meaningful to the user. DeWalt said he agreed and believed that Zikmund-Fisher's presentation raised the right points. He said it was important to recognize, however, that when a clinician or a tool says that a risk is high that a value is being placed on that risk. He noted that different people have different perspectives on whether a risk value is high, and that one of the most difficult things to do as a provider is to elicit a patient's values. Many providers will follow the guidelines, which for cardiovascular disease set 10 percent as high risk, DeWalt said. He gave as an example a risk calculator that is used at his clinic with which the patient's risk number turns red when it reaches 10 percent. This is effective at getting the patient's attention and prompting action. Patients whose risk is at 9 percent are not as motivated, yet there is little practical difference between 9 and 10 percent.

Zikmund-Fisher responded that he agreed that whenever underlying data are categorized, a value judgment is being imposed as to what differences and thresholds are meaningful and what ethical questions arise from this. Not providing the categorization, however, is also an ethical choice, Zikmund-Fisher noted. It is a choice to leave the recipient of the number without any context or knowledge of how to interpret that number. Zikmund-Fisher said the question of patient values is reflected in the signal being given. Framing the result as a signal to talk to one's doctor is qualitatively different from framing it as a signal to act. Zikmund-Fisher noted that not all labels are equivalent and there are different ways to group or categorize information for certain circumstances. It is important to ask what task people are being asked to do. Are they being asked to have the self-concept of a person with high risk? Or is the task to act or not to act? Conscious choices must be made about what people are being asked to do and how information is being presented, Zikmund-Fisher said.

Cindy Brach, roundtable member, commented that in developing the Health Literacy Universal Precautions Toolkit, she and DeWalt struggled with the most effective way to communicate test and laboratory results to patients. In the end the method they chose was to tell people whether their results were high and, if they were, to consult a physician. She noted that this was an imperfect approach, but the only one that struck an appropriate balance between just giving information and actually providing people with the tools to interpret that information. The goal is to illuminate the meaning behind the number, but this can come at the expense of the conversation that the patient needs to have with the provider about personal preferences and notions of risk. Zikmund-Fisher responded that the conflict between how to simplify yet accurately reflect the complexity of risk is inherent in the problem. Providers and patients need to have a conversation about potential risks and benefits when there is no clear, simple answer. The signal that needs to be given is to have the conversation, not that there is a clear answer. Zikmund-Fisher gave as an example the question of when to stop routine cancer screenings. He said he would not want to define an absolute threshold, but there is a point at which mammograms and colonoscopies are no longer beneficial. He said he would like to develop a way to determine when having that conversation with a patient is appropriate, rather than a guideline for when to stop screening.

Linda Harris, roundtable member, commented that if patients and providers had substantive conversations about risk, then the number would matter far less to a patient's confidence that he or she had made the right decision. A relationship with a trusted, reliable person developed over time is going to make a bigger difference in whether people believe they have made good decisions. Zikmund-Fisher replied that he both agreed and disagreed with that statement. While there is value and importance in that relationship, he thinks that people are more trusting of a categorization or a recommendation if they know data are supporting it. A patient does not have to be given the data up front, but there are times when it is beneficial to see the numbers and have some context. Harris then asked, what kind of conversation should providers and patients be having? What is the design of that conversation? Zikmund-Fisher agreed and said that just because the information exists does not mean it is the best way to inform someone of their risk or actions that should be taken. Providers should ask themselves what needs to be communicated at that level; maybe it is the numbers and data or maybe it is a more qualitative communication.

Roundtable member Ruth Parker asked Krughoff about the lessons he has learned over the years from being involved in providing information about health plans and health choices to people in a way that helps consumers make good choices. She also asked how he and his organization solicited feedback from consumers with the goal of improving the process. Krughoff answered that one of the biggest lessons he has learned is that people care a great deal about cost comparison. He added that comparing the costs of health plans can be baffling, however, and must be made simpler to allow people to understand it. He said that when soliciting feedback from users, his organization would watch people as they used the health plan comparison tool, record what they do, and then talk to them about why they made the choices they did and what could be improved. He noted that when choosing which aspect of a health plan is most important, people will make very different choices in some areas, while other areas remain constant. The importance of coverage for specific diseases varies greatly, but the quality and availability of doctors is consistently important to people. Two options—whether the health plan helps its members choose the right treatment and whether the plan participates in coordination of care—are consistently rated as not important by consumers. Krughoff said he believes this is an area where better consumer education may help because health plans can play a big role in these areas, but consumers do not seem to be aware of that. Parker followed up by saying that the ability to understand costs was one of consumers' most pressing needs. Krughoff agreed and said that his organization has been involved in the development of two state health insurance exchanges and he has been shocked by how little attention has been paid to the ability of consumers to compare plans. It has been overshadowed by eligibility and enrollment concerns.

Wilma Alvarado-Little, roundtable member, asked if any accommodations were made in the Consumers' CHECKBOOK tool for consumers who are visually impaired, have limited English skills, or have other challenges to using the tool. Krughoff replied that not enough accommodations were available for users with disabilities or challenges. He said he hopes that states or the federal government would make funds available to implement necessary accommodation and that Consumers' CHECKBOOK would be happy to help make that happen.

Kim Parson, roundtable member, asked how long the Consumers' CHECKBOOK tool has been in use. Krughoff answered that the tool has been in use for 34 years. For the first 22 years, it was in book form, but for the past 12 years, it has been available online. Many federal agencies subscribe to it for their employees. Parson then asked whether consumers have been satisfied with the tool and whether it has helped people to make better choices. Krughoff replied that the consumer satisfaction feedback they receive is very good; people have been very happy with the tool. Consumers' CHECKBOOK follows up with consumers about their choices by asking what plan they had, what plan they currently have, and why they made that choice. He said the appropriate choice question is heavily weighted toward cost. Although the organization may think a consumer made the wrong choice, he said it might not be wrong for that consumer. It is important to ask people why they chose as they did and compare their choices to what they say they care about. He added that Consumers' CHECKBOOK tries to get feedback and learn from it and that he does think the tool is helpful.

Roundtable member Linda Harris asked if Consumers' CHECKBOOK would be providing a tool for the health insurance marketplaces. Krughoff said the organization had written a paper on what should be included in the marketplaces to help consumers choose between plans.[4] The paper has had some positive response. Krughoff said that right now people are preoccupied with the mechanics of the marketplaces, and helping consumers choose has not been a priority. He said he thinks it will come eventually, but not when the marketplaces first open, unfortunately. Consumers' CHECKBOOK is developing a provider directory for one state and has been able to access the U.S. Department of Health and Human Services' physician

---

[4] The paper is available at http://www.checkbook.org/exchange/Health%20plan%20comparison%20tool--best%20practices%20recommendations.pdf (accessed October 29, 2013).

comparison website for that project. He noted that a consumer organization may have access to information that others do not and the credibility to make the system better.

Margaret Loveland, roundtable member, commented that the workshop highlighted that numeracy affects everyone. She added that health care providers and professionals can partner with journalists and consumers to communicate more clearly and that education must play a larger role in helping people develop better numeracy skills. She concluded by saying that ethics must be ingrained into everything a health professional does and that providers should not use their opinions to influence patients instead of giving them the facts.

Lindsey Robinson, roundtable member, commented that oral health was not highlighted in the workshop, but that it is important with regard to health literacy and numeracy. The oral cavity is the gateway into the gastrointestinal system and the entire body. She added that the concept of translating information and communicating effectively with patients and consumers can best be expressed in terms of keeping it simple so that people can understand.

Another roundtable member, Steven Rush, said it was energizing to hear about the research being undertaken on numeracy and cognitive skills. The challenge is how to move from thinking that health literacy is based on reading skills to realizing that health literacy is also math skills and cognitive processing skills when the focus has been on grade-level reading skills for some time.

Laurie Francis, roundtable member, found the workshop to be an important reminder that health literacy is bidirectional. It is a combination of both the communicator and the patient or consumer. A person may have low health literacy, but the provider may have low communication skills. It is important to teach providers and the entire team of people who work around the patient to communicate well. She noted that it was exciting to consider taking this concept outside of the medical model and that it is intriguing to think that health information technology can play a role in helping providers and patients communicate better.

Wilma Alvarado-Little, roundtable member, asserted that there are a number of urgent tasks related to health literacy and numeracy. Education is key to increasing numeracy and cognitive processing skills. Alvarado-Little said that youth are not being taught math to use in real-world situations and that there is a disconnect between education and real-world skills. She added that numeracy must also be part of the conversation regarding health insurance exchanges, navigators, and community-based organizations that are working to help people obtain health insurance.

Cindy Brach, roundtable member, commented that it was gratifying to learn that Consumers' CHECKBOOK is using Agency for Healthcare

Research and Quality data from the Medical Expenditure Panel Survey and the Consumer Assessment of Healthcare Providers and Systems surveys to help people make real-world decisions about their health coverage. She added that she spends a great deal of time focusing on reducing the demands of the system for health literacy and that there is not very good science on reducing the cognitive demands for quantitative information. This is not a call for more research, said Brach, but rather an endorsement of a universal precautions approach to health literacy. This is particularly important when considering that evidence shows that people will often say they understand the information, but when asked to demonstrate that understanding, they cannot. It is important to use methods like teach-back all the time because the question of how to communicate quantitative information effectively has not been answered. In addition, Brach said, it is disheartening to hear about the poor state of math skills and math teaching in the schools. She worries that it will lead to a further retreat from subjects such as art, music, and physical education. This should be a call for education to include those math skills in the teaching of other subjects rather than to forego those subjects in favor of further math drills.

Terri Parnell, roundtable member, said the workshop reminded her of the burden that numeracy interpretation places on health and treatment decision making, especially for areas such as end-of-life and palliative care as well as outcomes and costs. The discussion was energizing, she said, and led her to start thinking of ways to use numeracy to engage and empower patients and consumers.

Susan Pisano, roundtable member, expressed a need for a summary of the principles for good approaches to numeracy and icons and for the overall issues of numeracy. She noted that she found Apter's tool for helping providers communicate better with their patients to be particularly helpful.

Ruth Parker, roundtable member, commented that just as much of literacy is beyond words, numeracy with regard to cost is beyond numbers. Transparency in costs and helping people understand costs will require a culture shift in health care and new language and approaches. She noted that people are not given the price of an airline ticket when they arrive at their destination, but that is what happens in health care. Changing this approach will be an enormous change for both providers and consumers, but it is key to helping people understand and make decisions about their health care. Parker said she also believes it is time for health literacy professionals to build meaningful relationships with those who communicate in journalism and social media.

Another roundtable member, Gemirald Daus, said it is important to consider numeracy and literacy separately. Separating the two sets of skills will help to conceptualize the challenges that people will face with the ACA and the health insurance exchanges, in particular with the infrastructure that will be required to help people choose a health insurance plan. A significant proportion of new health care consumers may be from traditionally disadvantaged groups such as racial and ethnic minorities and those at low socioeconomic levels. The guidance and resources that are put toward enrolling people in health insurance plans must confront the challenges of low numeracy skills directly.

George Isham, roundtable member, commented that he was interested in the earlier conversation about the meaning of numbers in risk communication. The magnitude of the problem of communicating health information is enormous when one takes into consideration low health numeracy and the number of tasks that require numeracy skills, from preventive and medical care decision making to daily tasks of medication management. The evidence presented at the workshop shows that a large proportion of the millions of people engaged in those tasks will have trouble performing them due to a limited understanding of the numbers involved. In the short term, this problem will not be solved by better education, Isham added, but by focusing on decision architectures for common decisions and reducing demands on the patient. Education is very important in the long term but, given the magnitude of the problem, is not a solution for the next few decades. Physicians will need help with the process engineering that will help patients make more informed decisions. There are many compelling examples of decision making in contemporary American medicine, Isham said, that are wrong from the standpoint of use and misuse in which professionals have been silently complicit. This raises the ethical issue because there is a question as to the proper role for the medical professional in patient decision making.

Linda Harris, roundtable member, observed there seems to be a paradox at work with regard to numbers, precision, and decision making. That is, the more precise the number given, the less informative it tends to be for the patient. Reducing complexity is not enough; health communication must be focused on the interaction because that allows for embracing the complexity and finding ways to communicate it. Harris also asked about the ethics of giving a patient a number and not giving them the opportunity to have a meaningful conversation with a provider about it.

Jill Griffiths, roundtable member, commented that as vice president for communications at Aetna, she speaks to reporters every day who are looking for information on the ACA. There is a need and an opportunity within the fields of both journalism and health literacy to build a stronger partnership, and that is an area where the roundtable can be helpful. She added that two of the graphics in the speaker presentations were two different triangles representing the relationships between doctors, patients, and information and doctors, patients, and pharmacists. She asked if it was possible that these relationships could be merged together to create a different paradigm. This possibility creates significant opportunities to improve patient and consumer understanding.

Lori Hall, roundtable member, noted that context has been a recurrent theme from speakers at roundtable workshops. Bridget McCandless, a speaker at the Organizational Change to Improve Health Literacy workshop on April 11, 2013, spoke eloquently on the need to frame conversations about health and risk in ways that are relevant to patients. McCandless said that her patients were primarily low-income individuals living paycheck to paycheck and that she had found it was more useful to talk to them about the short-term consequences of poor health than the long-term consequences. Hall said that low numeracy skills in the population bring about a similar circumstance and highlight the importance of communicating risk in a language that is meaningful to the audience. Hall added that from a pharmaceutical industry perspective, it is important to note that numeracy skills are often measured in healthy individuals. When a person is sick or under stress, however, even those with the highest skill levels can struggle to understand the information they are being given. This is parallel to a phenomenon seen in clinical trials, Hall said. A patient's experience with a medication regime in a clinical trial is very controlled. Once the medication is on the market, the evidence from the real world may not match the evidence from the clinical trial because people are taking the medication under different circumstances, when they are under stress and do not have the same support as in the clinical trial. This highlights a challenge faced by the pharmaceutical industry with regard to representing risk and providing information to consumers. The language that pharmaceutical companies use to communicate risk is limited by the regulatory environment. It is very difficult to provide plain-language information to consumers. Hall said she believes this could be a topic for a future workshop.

Kim Parson, roundtable member, said numeracy adds another level of complexity to health and health care. She challenged the roundtable as a group to look for opportunities to partner with consumers and work to simplify this complex system.

Patrick McGarry, roundtable member, commented that numeracy is one of the greatest health literacy challenges. This workshop underscored the importance of numeracy and patient education, particularly the concept that the way information is conveyed must take into account the patient's specific and immediate needs. He added that he agreed there are important ethical considerations in the debate between when it is appropriate to present data to inform or to persuade.

Roundtable member Rima Rudd agreed that numeracy is a central issue of health literacy. Numeracy is important not just to understanding, but is also central to decision making. Rudd noted that many of the presentations were a reminder of the importance of scholarship and rigor in health literacy work. The most successful interventions were those that were piloted and rigorously examined. It is also important to form partnerships with other disciplines; health literacy professionals can do much more when they partner with communication or numeracy experts. That there are many adults with poor literacy and numeracy skills is not new information, Rudd said. She remarked that it is no longer an ethical dilemma on how to communicate effectively with patients and consumers, but an ethical imperative to learn how to do so. It is unethical to continue to make such huge demands on people when it is known that they are not able to meet them.

Darren DeWalt, roundtable member, noted that numbers are ubiquitous and that everyone faces challenges in understanding them at certain times. The solution to the problems of low numeracy skills is the same as many other health literacy problems: reduce complexity. There are some tools for accomplishing that that are specific to numbers, but the general concept is the same. It must be allowed, however, that there is complexity that must be faced and addressed in a conversation with a provider. Finally, DeWalt said, it is important to remember the task when designing a tool. Often things are designed in a way that does not take into account the task that the person using it must accomplish.

Robert Logan of the National Library of Medicine (NLM) commented that the question is how to help people make sense of the huge amount of information available to them. He noted that the NLM has created a database with summaries of clinical trials in a standardized format. Making this information available to the public was the result of a massive effort that took years to complete. It is important, however, to realize the work is not done. The fact that the information is available does not make it understandable and useful. People, including patients and providers, need to be taught how to use these kinds of resources that are becoming more and more available to them.

Benard Dreyer, roundtable member, agreed that numeracy is a critical issue in health literacy. Numeracy skills are very low in the general population. Even if a person is measured as proficient, he or she will probably still struggle with numeracy in times of illness or stress. In addition, health care professionals are not always proficient in numeracy and must be better trained and educated in numbers and communicating numbers. Dreyer added that in his opinion, there is a need to make information meaningful by categorizing and evaluating it for the patient or consumer. The complexity of the data can be addressed for people who would like that, but it should not be required for making decisions.

Transparency adds to trust and secrecy adds to mistrust, asserted roundtable member Paul Schyve. People trust their physicians when they believe there is transparency in their communication. Sometimes simply having the information available where an individual can access it if he or she desires creates this trust. Many things in society are becoming more complex, and numeracy plays a part in that, whether an individual is working in a factory or a restaurant. However, addressing this complexity is particularly urgent for the health care system because it affects lives and health. Schyve concluded by saying there is a lot to learn about improving communication and numeracy from fields outside of health care, and as professionals within the health care system learn and adjust, they can help to address the larger societal issues.

Schyve concluded the day by thanking the presenters and roundtable members for a fascinating and informative workshop.

## REFERENCES

Davis, T. C., M. S. Wolf, P. F. Bass, 3rd, J. A. Thompson, H. H. Tilson, M. Neuberger, and R. M. Parker. 2006. Literacy and misunderstanding prescription drug labels. *Annals of Internal Medicine* 145(12):887-894.

Hsee, C. K. 1996. The evaluability hypothesis: An explanation for preference reversals between joint and separate evaluations of alternatives. *Organizational Behavior and Human Decision Processes* 67(3):247-257.

Witteman, H. O., B. J. Zikmund-Fisher, E. A. Waters, T. Gavaruzzi, and A. Fagerlin. 2011. Risk estimates from an online risk calculator are more believable and recalled better when expressed as integers. *Journal of Medical Internet Research* 13(3):e54.

Wolf, M. 2013. *Effectively communicating medication instructions.* Presentation at the Institute of Medicine Workshop on Health Literacy and Numeracy, Washington, DC, July 18.

Yin, H. S., B. P. Dreyer, L. van Schaick, G. L. Foltin, C. Dinglas, and A. L. Mendelsohn. 2008. Randomized controlled trial of a pictogram-based intervention to reduce liquid medication dosing errors and improve adherence among caregivers of young children. *Archives of Pediatric and Adolescent Medicine* 162(9):814-822.

Zikmund-Fisher, B. J. 2013a. *Communicating quantitative decision making.* Presentation at the Institute of Medicine Workshop on Health Literacy and Numeracy, Washington, DC, July 18.

Zikmund-Fisher, B. J. 2013b. The right tool is what they need, not what we have: A taxonomy of appropriate levels of precision in patient risk communication. *Medical Care Research and Review* 70(Suppl 1):37S-49S.

Zikmund-Fisher, B. J., M. Dickson, and H. O. Witteman. 2011. Cool but counterproductive: Interactive web-based risk communications can backfire. *Journal of Medical Internet Research* 13(3):e60.

# Appendix A

# Numeracy and the Affordable Care Act: Opportunities and Challenges[1]

*Ellen Peters, Louise Meilleur, and Mary Kate Tompkins,*
*Psychology Department, Ohio State University*

## ABSTRACT

*Numbers are used to instruct, inform, and give meaning to information in order to help us make better judgments and healthier choices in our everyday lives. However, research has demonstrated that not all people can understand and use numbers effectively. In particular, people differ in numeracy. Among uninsured adults, we estimated that 28.8 percent are at a Below Basic level of numeracy, 33.4 percent are at a Basic level, 29.3 percent are at an Intermediate level, and only 8.6 percent are at a Proficient level of numeric literacy. Numeracy skills needed to select a health plan, choose treatments, and understand medication instructions include education-based skills and emergent decision-based abilities. We estimate that the skills needed to make many complex, informed health decisions (e.g., management of chronic diseases) require a Proficient level of numeric literacy, given how numeric information is often provided. However, if health information providers present information to patients and consumers in an evidence-based manner, a greater proportion of the population will be successful in making informed health and health-related decisions. We identify five main communication themes and discuss evidence-based strategies for communication under each theme.*

---

[1]Paper commissioned by the Roundtable on Health Literacy, Institute of Medicine.

## INTRODUCTION

Numbers are used to instruct, inform, and give meaning to information in order to help us make better judgments and healthier choices in our everyday lives. However, research has demonstrated that not all people can understand and use numbers effectively. In particular, people differ in numeracy. Numeracy has been variously defined as the ability to use basic probability and mathematical concepts (Peters et al., 2006b) and as "the degree to which individuals can obtain, process, and understand the basic [quantitative] health information and services they need to make appropriate health decisions" (Ratzan and Parker, 2000, p. vi). Berkman et al. (2011, p. 1) further describe the concept of health numeracy as representing "a constellation of skills necessary to function effectively in the health care environment and act appropriately on health care information." Even highly educated individuals can be innumerate (Lipkus et al., 2001).

Previous reports have focused on what is known about the relation of numeracy to health outcomes and disparities (Berkman et al., 2011). With so many Americans lacking basic numeracy skills, it is important to know whether and how numeracy influences health outcomes and health disparities. Berkman et al. (2011) conducted a systematic review of numeracy. They concluded that the strength of current evidence was insufficient with respect to the relation of numeracy to health outcomes such as knowledge, risk perception accuracy, and accurate interpretation of health information. Numeracy, however, did appear to mediate some health disparities (e.g., between race and levels of hemoglobin A1c and between gender and HIV medication management capacity), although the strength of evidence was low. Conclusions could not be drawn about the relation of numeracy to use of health care services. Numeracy does appear to be more highly correlated with health outcomes than is health literacy, although possible ceiling effects on health literacy could have clouded the health literacy effects.

In the present commissioned paper, our assignment was to consider the following statement of task: "With the implementation of health care reform, there will be an influx of previously uncovered individuals who have limited knowledge, understanding, and ability to navigate the health care choices available. Of particular importance will be numeracy skills needed to make informed choices about which health plan best meets individual needs, how to make informed treatment decisions (e.g., X treatment has a 5 percent greater risk than Y), and understanding medication instructions. The roundtable will hold a meeting July 18, 2013, in Washington, DC, to explore such issues."

This commissioned paper addresses three questions:

1. What does research show about people's numeracy skill levels?
2. What kinds of numeracy skills are needed to select a health plan, choose treatments, and understand medication instructions?
3. How can providers communicate with those with low numeracy skills?

## QUESTION 1: WHAT DOES RESEARCH SHOW ABOUT PEOPLE'S NUMERACY SKILL LEVELS?

Numeracy can be assessed with objective measures (e.g., "If person A's chance of getting a disease is 1 in 100 in 10 years and person B's risk is double that of A, what is B's risk?") (Cokely et al., 2012; Lipkus et al., 2001; Weller et al., 2013) and subjective measures (e.g., "How good are you at working with fractions?") (Fagerlin et al., 2007b). There are also general health numeracy measures, such as the Numeracy Understanding in Medicine instrument (NUMi) (Shapira et al., 2012) and various numeracy measures specific to health domains such as asthma, diabetes, and anti-coagulation control (Apter et al., 2006; Estrada et al., 2004; Huizinga et al., 2008). Other studies have simply tallied how well individuals can do specific health-related numeric tasks. For example, in an online survey representative of the U.S. population, 79 percent of parents claimed to have seen a growth chart before, and most think they understand them well (Ben-Joseph et al., 2009). However, when provided with multiple-choice questions and answers, only 64 percent could identify a child's weight when shown a plotted point on a growth chart and up to 77 percent misinterpreted charts that included both height and weight measurements. Like other innumeracy-related health examples, this may be important because parents may use their (inaccurate) understanding to guide related health decisions for their children.

As suggested above, Americans have limited numeracy skills. A recent probabilistic sample of Americans answered fewer than two-thirds of simple statistical numeracy questions correctly (Galesic and Garcia-Retamero, 2010). Even for the easiest question ("If the chance of getting a disease is 10 percent, how many people would be expected to get the disease out of 1,000?"), 17 percent answered incorrectly. For the most difficult item ("In the Daily Times Sweepstakes, the chance of winning a car is 1 in 1,000. What percentage of tickets for the Daily Times Sweepstakes win a car?"), participants had to translate 1 in 1,000 to a percentage; only 24 percent did so successfully. Wide disparities in numeracy also existed such that higher scores existed for men versus women, younger adults versus older adults, more educated adults versus less educated adults, and higher versus lower income adults (independent effects existed for only sex, education, and income).

The 2003 National Assessment of Adult Literacy (NAAL) defined numeracy (also called quantitative literacy) as "the ability to understand and use numbers in daily life" (Kutner et al., 2007). They estimated the proportion of Americans who fall into Below Basic, Basic, Intermediate, and Proficient quantitative literacy performance levels. The survey was administered to more than 19,000 adults (ages 16 and older) living in households or prisons. To be classified into each quantitative literacy level, one has to exhibit a set of specific quantitative skills and not exhibit the specific skills of the quantitative literacy level above it.

Key abilities that adults needed to demonstrate to be classified into each level can be found in Table A-1. For example, key abilities at the Below Basic level include finding numbers and using them to perform simple operations (mostly addition) when the information is familiar and concrete. For example, adding two numbers to complete an ATM deposit slip is a task categorized at the Below Basic level of quantitative literacy. In contrast, a sample task from the Intermediate level involved determining what time a person can take a prescription medication, given instructions on taking the medication in relation to eating. A sample task at the highest performance level, Proficient, involved calculating the yearly cost of life insurance using a table that gives the cost per month for each $1,000 of coverage. Individuals with less than Proficient abilities (those at Below Basic, Basic, or Intermediate levels) are expected not to be able to perform this sample life insurance task.

Results from the NAAL indicated that 22 percent of American adults are at the Below Basic level, 33 percent are at the Basic level, 33 percent are at the Intermediate level, and 13 percent are at the Proficient level of quantitative literacy. Results also indicated demographic differences

**TABLE A-1** Key Abilities and Estimated Proportion of Adults at Each Level of Quantitative Literacy

| Quantitative Literacy Level | % of Adults in Each Level (NAAL findings) | Estimated % (#) of Uninsured Adults in Each Level* | Estimated % (#) of Insured Adults in Each Level* | Key Abilities Associated with Level (NAAL) |
|---|---|---|---|---|
| Below Basic | 22% | 28.8% or 9,169,063 | 18.2% or 30,596,144 | Locating numbers and using them to perform simple quantitative operations (primarily addition) when the mathematical information is very concrete and familiar |

## TABLE A-1 Continued

| Quantitative Literacy Level | % of Adults in Each Level (NAAL findings) | Estimated % (#) of Uninsured Adults in Each Level* | Estimated % (#) of Insured Adults in Each Level* | Key Abilities Associated with Level (NAAL) |
|---|---|---|---|---|
| Basic | 33% | 33.4% or 10,656,748 | 31.9% or 53,702,419 | Locating easily identifiable quantitative information and using it to solve simple, one-step problems when the arithmetic operation is specified or easily inferred |
| Intermediate | 33% | 29.3% or 9,339,640 | 35.3% or 59,508,631 | Locating less familiar quantitative information and using it to solve problems when the arithmetic operation is not specified or easily inferred |
| Proficient | 13% | 8.6% or 2,749,954 | 14.6% or 24,505,031 | Locating more abstract quantitative information and using it to solve multistep problems when the arithmetic operations are not easily inferred and the problems are more complex |
| Total U.S. Population 200,227,629 | 101% | 100.1% or 31,915,404 | 100% or 168,312,225 | |

NOTE: Individuals at each level of quantitative literacy are thought to have the skills identified at that level, but are thought to not have the skills at levels above their own (e.g., an individual with Below Basic quantitative literacy should have the skills located in that row, but would not have the skills located in the rows for Basic, Intermediate, or Proficient literacy).

* These estimates are not based on perfectly comparable samples. The sample from the NAAL consists of people ages 16 years and older living in households or prisons whereas the sample from the 2009-2011 Census is a civilian noninstitutionalized population 25 years and over. Both samples also include older adults (65 years and older) who are not as relevant to Patient Protection and Affordable Care Act concerns because most are covered by Medicare. Although older adults tend to be less numerate, their inclusion likely affects the uninsured estimates very little (because most are insured), but means that the insured population of younger individuals 18 to 64 years old likely has higher quantitative skills than reflected in Table A-1.

in quantitative abilities. Males scored higher than females, high-income individuals scored higher than low income, and the more educated scored higher than the less educated. In addition, scores among white and Asian/Pacific Islander adults were higher than scores for black and Hispanic adults. No analyses were available concerning whether any single demographic variable predicted quantitative literacy scores over and above other demographic variables.

The proportions of individuals at each quantitative literacy level are based on the overall U.S. population, however, and may not accurately reflect the numeracy abilities we should expect from previously uninsured adults who will now enter the health care system as the result of the Patient Protection and Affordable Care Act (ACA). By combining the NAAL data with the 2009-2011 Census Bureau data (U.S. Census Bureau, 2009-2011), we estimated the proportion of uninsured and insured American adults who fall into Below Basic, Basic, Intermediate, and Proficient quantitative literacy categories (see Table A-1). For these estimates, we used the 2003 NAAL that provides data on the proportion of adults in each quantitative literacy level based on their educational attainment; the Census Bureau (2009-2011) provides data on the proportion of uninsured and insured adults at each level of educational attainment.

Using these two data sources, we estimated that *among uninsured adults* 28.8 percent are at the Below Basic level, 33.4 percent are at the Basic level, 29.3 percent are at the Intermediate level, and only 8.6 percent are at the Proficient level. *Among insured adults*, we estimated that 18.2 percent are at the Below Basic level, 31.9 percent are at the Basic level, 35.3 percent are at the Intermediate level, and 14.6 percent are at the Proficient level. See Table Annex A-1 in this appendix for a more detailed explanation of how these estimates were calculated and the limitations of these estimates. Given these estimates, roughly 29 percent (9,170,000) of uninsured adults and 18 percent (30,600,000) of insured adults lack the Basic quantitative skills necessary to locate quantitative information and use it to solve simple one-step arithmetic problems. Approximately 62 percent (19,800,000) of uninsured adults and 50 percent (84,300,000) of insured American adults lack the Intermediate quantitative skills necessary to locate less familiar quantitative information and use it to solve problems in which the arithmetic operation is not specified.

### Dual-Process Theories and the Potential Influence of Time Pressure, Stress, and Illness on Reductions to Health Numeracy Skills

Research in numeracy has been associated with what are known as "dual-process theories" in decision making (Peters et al., 2006b). Information in decision making appears to be processed using an analytic mode of thinking and an affective/experiential one (Epstein, 1994; Loewenstein et al., 2001; Reyna, 2004; Sloman, 1996; also called Systems 1 and 2, respectively, Kahneman, 2003; Stanovich and West, 2002). In particular, numeracy is considered an analytical skill—one has to think to do number calculations. Both modes of thought are important to forming decisions. The experiential mode is primarily based on affective (emotional) feelings, and processing using this mode is relatively effortless, automatic, and spontaneous. As shown in a number of studies, the affective feelings that are primary to this mode of thought provide both meaning and motivation to choice processes (Damasio, 1994). Processing in the analytic mode, on the other hand, is conscious, deliberative, reason based, verbal, and relatively slow. The analytical mode of thinking is more flexible and provides effortful control over more spontaneous experiential processes. Both modes of thinking are important and good choices are most likely to emerge when affective and analytical modes work in concert and decision makers think as well as feel their way through judgments and decisions (Damasio, 1994). Research, however, has demonstrated that the experiential mode (and affect, in particular) has a relatively greater influence when analytical capacity is lower due to cognitive load or time pressure (Finucane et al., 2000; Shiv and Fedorikhin, 1999).

This distinction is important because being involved in health decisions often involves factors that reduce how well patients and consumers think (e.g., time pressure for a patient to make an informed choice in a physician's office, being sick, being stressed, or being overwhelmed with too much information). As a result, the numeric abilities of representative U.S. populations may overestimate the numeracy levels of patients making health decisions. This is because reported numeracy abilities for the U.S. population are usually measured in healthy individuals who are not under time pressure, whereas patients seen by health care providers may be subject to one of the factors above (e.g., being sick). These reduced numeracy abilities may lead to numeric sources of information being less well understood and used in health decisions, while less relevant sources of affect and emotion play a larger role. Little health research, however, exists concerning this possibility.

## QUESTION 2: WHAT KINDS OF NUMERACY SKILLS ARE NEEDED TO SELECT A HEALTH PLAN, CHOOSE TREATMENTS, AND UNDERSTAND MEDICATION INSTRUCTIONS?

### Education-Based Numeracy Skills

Apter and colleagues (2008) presented a hierarchy of mathematical skills required to successfully complete numeric tasks while making health decisions. Higher level tasks include estimation, understanding probabilities, problem solving (the ability to decipher when and how to apply a numerical skill), understanding variability and error in measurement, and risk assessment. See the education-based numeracy skills of Table A-2 adapted from Apter et al. (2008). Having the skills to successfully complete these tasks is expected to allow patients and consumers to locate numeric information and transform it in ways that allow them to make more effective decisions about their health. Education-based skills are divided into four main skill categories: basic, computational, analytical, and statistical numeric skills. The basic skill to understand numeric information is necessary for many health-related tasks. When choosing a health plan from a health insurance exchange, for example, consumers must be able to read and understand basic fees and use simple arithmetic operations, such as adding costs together. Such understanding is a fundamental building block to deciding which health plans they prefer and can afford. Similarly, taking medications correctly requires the ability to read and understand dosage and timing instructions. Computational skills to do tasks such as estimating sizes and understanding how to work with frequencies and percentages are particularly important when making treatment decisions because options can be described based on the likelihood of risks and benefits in frequentistic form (e.g., 10 out of 100 patients) or percentage form (e.g., 10 percent of patients).

For tasks requiring analytical skills, patients and consumers must be able to apply numeric information to solve problems, make inferences, and interact with complex displays of information such as tables, graphs, and maps. For example, understanding numeric information provided in formats such as frequencies and percentages may not, by itself, be sufficient for accurate risk perception. Peters et al. (2006b) demonstrated that less numerate individuals were susceptible to format effects, presumably because the less numerate, although they likely understood the numbers in the sense that they could repeat them back accurately, did not transform numbers from one format to another. Specifically, in Peters et al. (2011), experimenters presented participants with the likelihood of an adverse event from a prescribed medication either in a frequentistic format (10 of 100 patients get a bad blistering rash) or a probabilistic format (10 percent of 100 patients get a bad blistering rash). Both formats are normatively equivalent. The experimenters found that less numerate individuals perceived a greater risk of an adverse event when the likelihood estimate was described in a frequentistic format (10 of 100) than when it was described in a probabilistic format (10 percent of 100). By contrast, highly numerate individuals rated the level of risk as the same in each information format. Normatively, the frame of information should not change the risk perception judgment.

**TABLE A-2** Education-Based Numeracy Skills from Apter et al. (2008) and Emergent Decision-Based Numeracy Skills Adapted from Peters (2012)

|  | Skill Categories | Numeracy-Related Tasks |
|---|---|---|
| Education-based numeracy skills | Basic | Reading numbers, counting, telling time |
| | | Arithmetic operations |
| | | Estimation of size, trend |
| | Computational | Frequency |
| | | Percentage |
| | | Problem solving and inferring the mathematical concepts to be applied |
| | Analytical | Logic |
| | | Reading tables |
| | | Reading graphs |
| | | Reading maps |
| | | Estimating error, uncertainty, variability |
| | Statistical | Relative versus absolute |
| | | Risk (cumulative, relative, conditional) |
| Emergent decision-based numeracy skills | Information seeking | Seeking numeric information rather than avoiding it |
| | | Willingness to perform computation |
| | Attention | More likely to attend to numeric information in a complex display |
| | | Able to disregard irrelevant information presented with numeric information |
| | Memory | Recall numeric information from memory |
| | Information sensitivity | Sensitivity to numeric information sources |
| | | Sensitivity to non-numeric information sources when numeric sources are available |
| | Affective meaning | Derive affective meaning (i.e., a sense of goodness or badness) from numeric information. Note: Affect comes into play when developing preferences and making decisions. National Assessment of Adult Literacy comparison examples do not include choice |

In taking medications, other kinds of format issues appear. For example, with liquid medication, patients often use inaccurate measurement devices such as household spoons, and they often confuse teaspoons and tablespoons (Madlon-Kay and Mosch, 2000). In selecting health plans, consumers sometimes want to estimate annual costs. To do so correctly, they must transform some numbers (e.g., monthly premiums and biannual physician visits to annual) in order to add them to other numbers (e.g., annual deductibles). Such calculations require analytical skills and knowing how to apply numeric information to solve problems.

Finally, Apter includes concepts related to probabilistic reasoning in the Statistical skill category. This includes the understanding of variability and randomness, being able to evaluate relative versus absolute comparisons, and being able to compare different risk assessments (cumulative, relative, and conditional). Such skills are important because inclusion of preventive care services in plans offered in health exchanges means that the newly insured will need to choose between treatment options, and also choose whether or not to obtain preventive health screenings and treatments. To do so, consumers first must realize they are susceptible to a given disease (e.g., understand concepts of randomness and variability), and then understand the risks from the disease as well as the risk reduction from taking preventive steps (both relative and absolute risks). For example, imagine a patient who accurately understands that his risk of developing type 2 diabetes is greater based on the percent chance (probability) of developing disease at his current weight. He can then estimate how much his risk will be reduced with effortful changes to diet and exercise, and he can choose to develop healthier behaviors. He may also be better able to follow through on effective behaviors due to superior understanding of how to count calories or do other number-related tasks. In another example, imagine a 50-year-old woman with no family history of breast cancer. Although her known risk factors are low, if she is highly numerate, she may understand that the inherent variability and randomness of health risks still means she is at risk. Understanding that risk, she may be more likely to pursue recommended screening procedures.

Apter et al.'s hierarchy focuses on math education and the computational skills necessary to function in a complex environment. Table A-2 lists the education-based numeracy skills as discussed by Apter et al. (2008). With respect to the NAAL quantitative literacy levels (Below Basic, Basic, Intermediate, and Proficient), The skills in Table A-2 do not align directly with particular levels, but Apter et al. (2008) listed the education-based skills in order of difficulty from least to most difficult. Table A-2 also includes emergent decision-based numeracy skills adapted from Peters (2012). The two types of skills are separated by a dashed line in Tables A-2 through A-5 for clarity.

## Emergent Decision-Based Numeracy Skills

Berkman et al. (2011) concluded that having a theoretical basis to interventions was an important component of effective interventions to reduce health disparities. As a result, we briefly review what is known about the psychological theory underlying numeracy's relation to health decision making. It is thought that numeracy exerts its influence on health outcomes in part through its effects on health decision making (Peters, 2012; Reyna et al., 2009). Understanding these underlying mechanisms should help in the design of more effective interventions in the future.

Psychological research on numeracy and decision making indicates that numeracy is also associated with emergent decision-based abilities not formally taught in school (see emergent decision-based abilities in Table A-2). Previous research has shown that higher numeracy is related (not surprisingly) to more comprehension of provided numeric information in a variety of domains, but it is also associated with a greater likelihood to seek out, attend to, and remember numeric information. Higher numeracy has also been associated with more precise number-related affect, a greater sensitivity to numbers in judgments and decisions, and less influence of non-numerical information (Peters et al., 2012). Some emergent decision-based numeracy abilities (e.g., more numerate individuals are less susceptible to various framing effects) have previously been identified by Apter et al. (2006) as being part of education-based skills, so we leave them categorized as education-based skills.

To begin, the highly numerate appear to be more motivated with respect to numeric information; they are more likely to seek it out, whereas less numerate individuals may avoid numeric information (Ancker and Kaufman, 2007; Keller, 2011; Lipkus and Peters, 2009). Such information seeking (and lack of information avoidance) is important when choosing whether to find out about the likelihood of a disease such as breast cancer (and possibly be screened for it) or deciding whether to take a new medication that has less than certain benefits and may cause adverse events. Highly numerate individuals, for example, might be more likely to examine detailed consumer medication information to find out about possible side effects and their associated likelihoods. They may also be more likely to pursue information about how to minimize the likelihood of potential medication side effects (e.g., eating and exercise behaviors when taking Coumadin®). Second, when faced with a complex display of information, higher numeracy is associated with a greater likelihood of attending to provided numeric information (Keller, 2011), as well as a greater ability to ignore irrelevant information (e.g., hospital information not related to the quality of care it offers) (Peters et al., 2007b). In the case of choosing a health plan, less numerate individuals might seek out, attend to, and be

**TABLE A-3** Health Plan Selection: Example Tasks

| Quantitative Literacy Level | Comparative NAAL Item | Example Task: Health Plan Selection | Skill Categories (from Table A-2) |
|---|---|---|---|
| Below Basic<br><br>(28.8% of uninsured population) | Calculate the price difference between two appliances, using information in a table that includes price and other information about the appliances. | Compare and calculate the difference between monthly premiums of two plans. | Basic; Analytical<br><br>Information Seeking; Attention |
| Basic<br><br>(33.4% of uninsured population) | Calculate the cost of a sandwich and salad, using prices from a menu. | Select the health plan with the lowest cost based on the annual premium and annual deductible for a family. | Basic; Computational; Analytical<br><br>Information Seeking; Attention; Memory |
| Intermediate<br><br>(29.3% of uninsured population) | Calculate the cost of raising a child for 1 year in a family with a specified income, based on a newspaper article that provides the percentage of a typical family's budget that goes toward raising children. | Calculate the coinsurance cost of an emergency room visit bill for $500 from a table of different coinsurance rates. | Basic; Computational; Analytical<br><br>Information Seeking; Attention |
| Proficient<br><br>(8.6% of uninsured population) | Calculate an employee's share of health insurance costs for 1 year, using a table that shows how the employee's monthly cost varies with income and family size. | Estimate total annual cost of the health plan, including premiums, copays, and deductibles, based on expected health care needs (e.g., estimating costs due to chronic illnesses such as diabetes or asthma). | Basic; Computational; Analytical; Statistical<br><br>Information Seeking; Attention; Memory; Information Sensitivity |

**TABLE A-4** Treatment Selection: Example Tasks

| Performance Level | Comparative NAAL Item | Example Task: Treatment Selection | Skill Categories (from Table A-2) |
|---|---|---|---|
| Below Basic<br><br>(28.8% of uninsured population) | Compare two prices by identifying the appropriate number and subtracting. | Compare and calculate the difference in copay amounts between generic and name-brand prescription drugs. | Basic; Analytical<br><br>Information Seeking; Attention |
| Basic<br><br>(33.4% of uninsured population) | Perform a two-step calculation to find the cost of three baseball tickets, using an order form that gives the price of one ticket and the postage and handling charge. | Calculate the difference in percentages of patients who survive one treatment compared to another. | Basic; Computational; Analytical; Statistical<br><br>Information Seeking; Attention |
| Intermediate<br><br>(29.3% of uninsured population) | Calculate the cost of raising a child for 1 year in a family with a specified income, based on a newspaper article that provides the percentage of a typical family's budget that goes toward raising children. | Calculate the proportion of patients who will suffer at least one adverse event based on patient age and three possible adverse events (assume independence of adverse events). | Basic; Computational; Analytical<br><br>Information Seeking; Attention |
| Proficient<br><br>(8.6% of uninsured population) | Calculate the yearly cost of a specified amount of life insurance, using a table that gives cost by month for each $1,000 of coverage. | Calculate the 5-year risk of fracture from an osteoporosis medication for a female patient of a given age, using a table that gives annual risk for each gender by age group. | Basic; Computational; Analytical; Statistical<br><br>Information Seeking; Attention |

**TABLE A-5** Understanding Medication Instructions: Example Tasks

| Performance Level | Comparative NAAL Item | Example Task: Understanding Medication and Treatment Instructions | Skill Categories (from Table A-2) |
|---|---|---|---|
| Below Basic<br><br>(28.8% of uninsured population) | Calculate the change from a $20 bill after paying the amount on a receipt. | Locate the risks of different side effects for the medication. Identify which side effect is most likely to occur. | Basic; Computational; Analytical<br><br>Information Seeking; Attention |
| Basic<br><br>(33.4% of uninsured population) | Perform a two-step calculation to find the cost of three baseball tickets, using an order form that gives the price of one ticket and the postage and handling charge. | 24 pills remain in a bottle of prescription medication. If you take 2 pills per day and refilling a prescription can take up to 7 days, in how many days should you order a refill to make sure that you do not run out of your prescription? | Basic; Computational; Analytical<br><br>Information Seeking; Attention |
| Intermediate<br><br>(29.3% of uninsured population) | Determine what time a person can take a prescription medication, based on information on the prescription drug label that relates timing of medication to eating. | "The patient forgot to take this medicine before lunch at noon. What is the earliest time he can take it in the afternoon?<br><br>GARFIELD, Robert M.<br>Dr. LUBIN, Michael<br>DOXYCYCLINE 100MG<br>Take one tablet on an empty stomach 1 hour before a meal or 2 to 3 hours after a meal unless otherwise directed by your doctor." | Basic; Analytical<br><br>Information Seeking; Attention; Memory (if time of last meal was not provided) |

**TABLE A-5** Continued

| Performance Level | Comparative NAAL Item | Example Task: Understanding Medication and Treatment Instructions | Skill Categories (from Table A-2) |
|---|---|---|---|
| Proficient (8.6% of uninsured population) | Determine the number of units of flooring required to cover the floor in a room, when the area of the room is not evenly divisible by the units in which the flooring is sold. | Diabetes management— understanding glucose meter readings, interpreting sliding-scale regimes, titrating oral medications or insulin, adjusting insulin for carbohydrate content. (Note: This example is much more complex than any of the NAAL examples used, but it is a realistic example of what patients are required to do.) | Basic; Computational; Analytical<br><br>Information Seeking; Attention; Memory; Information Sensitivity; Affective Meaning |

more easily influenced by anecdotes that describe the friendliness of an insurance provider's staff (e.g., from a neighbor or in marketing materials). At the same time, they may fail to adequately attend to the large annual deductible or copays required by the plan. In one study, for example, less numerate participants could usually understand which consumer-directed health plan had the lowest monthly premiums (we estimate this task to require Below Basic ability), but only about a third of them were able to identify which health plan was better if the patient needed a lot of care (a more difficult task that likely requires at least Intermediate ability) (Greene et al., 2008).

Highly numerate individuals also remember numeric information better than the less numerate (Sagara, 2009). Such numeracy effects, however, may be greatest soon after learning health information, then lessen over time. Galesic and Garcia-Retamero (2011), for example, studied how well participants recalled the consequences of health-related behaviors, such as being overweight or exercising, and cardiovascular health. Such recall may be important to following through on recommended behaviors. They found that highly numerate individuals recalled the consequences of health-related behaviors better than the less numerate after 10 minutes. Memory for both groups had declined after 3 weeks, and no statistically significant memory differences existed between the groups at this later time point. Of course, even the short-term memory advantage could be helpful in following the complex treatment plans required in management of chronic diseases such as diabetes. In these cases, patients either have to remember pertinent numeric information (carbohydrate consumption, blood glucose levels, insulin doses, times administered, etc.) in order to take the next step in managing their disease effectively, or they have to be diligent about recording it in the moment.

Previous research also has shown that highly numerate individuals draw more precise affective meaning from numbers than less numerate individuals. Using a paradigm modified from Denes-Raj and Epstein (1994), Peters et al. (2006b) presented participants with drawings of two bowls of jellybeans with different numbers of red and white jellybeans. Participants were told to imagine they could pick one bean and they would win $5 if the bean they selected was red. The larger bowl of 100 jellybeans had a higher number, but a smaller proportion (9 in 100 or 9 percent) of red jellybeans than the smaller bowl. The smaller bowl of 10 jellybeans had one red jellybean and a larger proportion (1 in 10 or 10 percent) of red jellybeans. Both bowls had the objective percentage of colored jellybeans labeled under each bowl. Participants were asked which bowl they would prefer to choose from and how clear a feeling they had about the goodness or badness of the larger bowl's 9 percent chance of winning. Peters et al. (2006b) found that the less numerate were more likely to choose bowl A, the suboptimal choice, than were more numerate individuals. The reason for this difference appeared to be that highly numerate individuals developed more precise feelings about the 9 percent chance of winning than the less numerate.

Being able to derive affective meaning from numbers and number comparisons is important in a health environment to compare treatment effectiveness or health care costs. Individuals can have strong affective reactions to risk and other numeric information, and this affect appears to guide risk perceptions and decisions (Slovic et al., 2005; Zikmund-Fisher et al., 2010). Studies have shown that without affect, numbers are not used in judgment and choice (Bateman et al., 2007; Peters et al., 2006b). In one study, for example, Fagerlin and colleagues (2005b) found that women asked to estimate their risk of breast cancer tended to overestimate that risk. Then, when told their actual risk, these women appeared to draw affective meaning from the number comparison. Compared to women who had not estimated their own risk first, they were quite relieved and perceived their cancer risk as lower than when they were simply told their cancer risk without having made their own estimate first. This is important because it may help to explain why counseling women about breast cancer risks decreases screening compliance. Although numeracy was not explicitly studied, highly numerate women may be more likely to show this and similar effects. As a result, although having greater numeracy generally leads to superior judgments and decisions because they are more likely to attend to numbers and number comparisons and derive affective meaning to guide their choices (Peters et al., 2006b), the highly numerate may sometimes demonstrate worse judgments than the less numerate.

Perhaps because of their greater abilities to attend to numeric information and draw affective meaning from it, highly numerate individuals tend to show a greater sensitivity to numeric information in health compared to the less numerate. For example, Lipkus et al. (2010) presented women with early-stage breast cancer with their chances of being cancer free during the next 10 years under four preventive cancer treatment decisions. They found that more numerate patients were sensitive to differences in cancer-free survival estimates for the treatments (they perceived themselves, on average, as more likely to survive when provided higher survival chances such as 92 percent than lower chances such as 63 percent); perceptions of the less numerate patients were almost completely insensitive to these same differences in survival odds. Among the women with the highest provided survival odds (average survival odds were about 92 percent), the less numerate were very pessimistic and perceived their 10-year survival odds as quite low on average (less than 45 percent); the highly numerate were also pessimistic, but perceived their odds as considerably higher (more than 75 percent).

The differences in sensitivity to numbers may also cause (or be caused by; the research is not clear on this point) an opposing difference in sensitivity to non-numeric information. In contrast to the highly numerate, less numerate individuals have shown a greater sensitivity to non-numeric and often emotional sources of information such as provided information frames (survival versus mortality rates are potential sources of emotion) and current mood states. In a study by Västfjäll and colleagues (in preparation), researchers manipulated participants' moods to be either positive or negative using a presumably unrelated recall task, and then asked participants to price a lottery ticket. Results indicated that less numerate participants were more influenced by the mood induction than highly numerate participants. In particular, the less numerate participants set higher prices for the lottery ticket in the positive-mood condition than the negative-mood condition. This is important because patients and consumers make many health judgments and decisions while in emotional states (e.g., the joy of a positive result; the anxiety of a new diagnosis). In Peters et al. (2009), less numerate participants also relied on their moods to judge the quality of care of a hospital rather than using provided numeric quality-of-care indicators;

the highly numerate used some of the provided numeric information and did not rely on their mood states in the moment.

Thus, previous research has shown that greater numeracy generally leads to better decision making. More numerate individuals tend to understand numbers better than the less numerate (and comprehension is a fundamental building block of good decisions). In addition, however, greater numeracy has been associated with a greater likelihood to seek out, attend to, and remember numeric information; to derive more precise number-related affect; to be more sensitive to numbers in judgments and decisions; and to be less influenced by non-numerical information (Peters, 2012). In general, the highly numerate do more work with numbers than do the less numerate, and these habits of the mind appear to coalesce and allow them to make superior number-based decisions.

The emergent decision-based abilities have not been linked explicitly with the four NAAL quantitative literacy levels. The extant research, however, supports these emergent abilities being present more among highly numerate individuals than the less numerate. As a result, individuals with higher levels of quantitative literacy will tend to exhibit more of these abilities. In particular, the emergent numeracy abilities are likely to be associated with either Intermediate or Proficient quantitative literacy levels. These abilities, however, can also emerge due to experience and/or motivation; individuals with lower numeracy will sometimes use these abilities nonetheless (e.g., seek out numeric information) if they have had experience in the health domain and understand its importance or if they are motivated in some other way (Hibbard et al., 2007b). Women, for example, although less numerate on average than men, often show what is likely a health care experience-based gender advantage (i.e., women tend to be more involved in family health decisions) (Ben-Joseph et al., 2009; Hibbard et al., 2007b).

Below we provide additional health examples in the three requested areas (following medication instructions, making health plan choices, and choosing treatments). We also attempt to match the examples, where possible, to the four levels of quantitative literacy identified in the NAAL to provide the reader with an idea of the approximate proportion of the previously uninsured population who will likely be able to do each task.

### Example Skills Needed to Select a Health Plan at Each Level of Quantitative Literacy

The ACA (section 1302) broadly defines the levels of coverage and the essential health benefits that must be included in new health insurance plans. It also leaves considerable room for variation between plans. Bronze, Silver, Gold, and Platinum plans must, respectively, cover 60, 70, 80, and 90 percent of the value of the benefits included in the plan, but a great deal of flexibility exists in how plans are implemented. Consumers are faced with financial decisions based on premiums, copayments, coinsurances, and annual deductibles. The broad definition of essential health benefits also allows for variation in the services covered, adding another layer of complexity to the decision process.

Table A-3 provides examples of tasks related to health plan selection that patients should be able to complete at each level of quantitative literacy. For each example, a comparative NAAL task is included for reference along with relevant skill categories from Table A-2 that we believe are needed to perform the task listed. Note that, as in Table A-2, the education-based skills and emergent decision-based skills are separated by a dashed line (education-based skills are above the dashed line in each row; emergent decision-based skills are below).

To make a health plan choice, consumers first must be able to locate and understand relevant pricing information. This initial task can be complicated by unfamiliarity with terms such as copay and coinsurance (Quincy, 2012). However, most consumers (even those with Below Basic ability) should be able to locate information, although one should keep in mind that the Below Basic group includes individuals with very low-level skills. In fact, previous attempts to assess how well younger and middle-aged adults locate cost and quality-of-care information in tables and charts indicate that about 9 percent errors might be expected even at this basic building block of the health plan selection process (Hibbard et al., 2001). It is not entirely clear how to adjust this finding for the group of previously uninsured individuals who will soon be making these choices, although the proportion of comprehension errors will be largest in the Below Basic group.

To compare different plans, consumers must be able to calculate differences in monthly premiums; this is expected to be a Below Basic skill that most consumers can perform successfully (see Table A-3 for the tasks and relevant skill categories). Selecting the health plan with the lowest cost based on the annual premium and deductible for a family is expected to be a Basic skill doable by about 71 percent of the uninsured population (everyone except those at the Below Basic level). With at least an Intermediate level of NAAL performance, more comprehensive evaluations of health plan costs are more likely, including calculations such as coinsurance costs based on a percentage of the cost of treatments. More complex calculations (e.g., calculating annual costs based on monthly premiums, estimated out-of-pocket expenses from flat-rate copayments, and estimated out-of-pocket expenses from percentage-based coinsurance amounts that meet annual deductibles), however, require much greater proficiency. Only an estimated 8.6 percent of the currently uninsured population is expected to have reached this Proficient quantitative literacy level. Moreover, consumers must be able to estimate their own future health care needs. For example, a patient with a chronic illness, such as asthma, needs multiple prescription drugs and may be best served by a plan with higher monthly premiums that covers a greater percentage of prescription drug costs. To determine which health plan best meets her needs, the patient must recall how much each prescription costs her and how many prescriptions she fills per year, add together the cost of these prescriptions, calculate the annual premium amount, and then calculate total costs for each plan and compare the total cost across multiple plan offerings. This is also expected to require Proficient quantitative literacy. Given the small proportion of individuals at the Proficient level in both the insured and uninsured groups (see Table A-1), it is not surprising that researchers have found consumers to be anxious, confused, and overwhelmed when making health plan choices (Day and Nadash, 2012; Quincy, 2012).

Beyond the difficulties posed in making the calculations to compare different health plans, individuals with Below Basic performance may be more prone than other individuals to focus on the most salient cost involved in health insurance, which, based on an analysis of Medicare Part D choices, is likely to be monthly premiums rather than out-of-pocket expenses (Abaluck and Gruber, 2011). Such patients may simply choose the plan with the lowest premium, not understanding that their total annual cost of services may be much higher than another plan with only slightly higher premiums (see also Greene et al., 2008).

## Example Skills Needed to Select Treatments at Each Level of Quantitative Literacy

Although decisions among health plans may rely largely on price calculations and comparisons, the decision of which treatment to choose is much less likely to include price as a component. This difference is primarily due to the ambiguity and variability of treatment costs and difficulty in obtaining them. Patients frequently do not receive cost information before treatments are administered (and may find out about or pay attention to only their portion of the costs afterward). Moreover, recent data highlighted the extreme price variability that exists among hospitals for similar treatments (CMS, 2013). As a result, even when patients want to evaluate treatment cost differences, accurate cost information can be complicated and difficult to obtain (Rosenthal et al., 2013). Treatment decisions tend to be based instead on the health care provider's recommendation and (when patients share in the decision) on the convenience of administration, medication copayments, and perceived risks and benefits of treatment options.

Table A-4 provides example NAAL tasks paired with treatment decision tasks estimated to fall into each performance level of quantitative literacy; relevant skill categories are also included. As in previous tables, the education-based skills and emergent decision-based skills are separated by a dashed line (education-based skills above, emergent decision-based skills below). Because the NAAL examples focus heavily on calculations of costs, the examples are not directly matched with our treatment option example tasks. In each example, the patient must be able and willing to seek out numeric information and attend to it; such ability and willingness could be derived from numeracy skills or from a motivation to care for the self or others (e.g., patient activation) (Hibbard et al., 2007a). Most patients, including those with Below Basic performance, likely will be able to compare the copay amounts between a generic and name-brand prescription drug. With at least a Basic level of quantitative literacy (an estimated 71.2 percent of the uninsured population), patients should be able to calculate the difference in survival rates between two treatment options when provided with the percentage of patients who survive. Having at least Intermediate quantitative literacy (an estimated 37.9 percent of the uninsured) would be necessary to complete a medication cost comparison based on the recommended dosage and unit cost of a medication (e.g., comparing the number of pills per dose and cost per pill in generic acetaminophen versus Tylenol in order to choose the less expensive option). Only those with Proficient quantitative skills (an estimated 8.6 percent of the uninsured) are expected to be able to calculate cumulative risks and benefits of treatments accurately and compare them to make treatment decisions based on trade-offs that are acceptable to them. For example, a woman with osteopenia might be advised to take a bisphosphonate for 3 to 5 years, but must choose whether or not to take it based on information about annual rates of risks and benefits.

### Example Skills Needed to Understand Medication Instructions at Each Level of Quantitative Literacy

Properly following medication instructions can be a difficult task for some patients (e.g., taking a prescription drug in their own homes). Although prescription drugs are labeled with dosage instructions, patients must be able to read and understand them, remember what time to take any medication, determine how to handle inadvertently missed doses, and, when appropriate, determine when to have prescriptions refilled to avoid running out of daily medications.

Table A-5 provides examples of the skills needed to follow medication and treatment instructions at each level of quantitative literacy performance, a comparative NAAL example, and relevant skill categories. Note that, as in Table A-2, the education-based skills and emergent decision-based skills are separated by a dashed line (education-based skills above, emergent decision-based skills below). Individuals with Below Basic abilities can be expected to locate the risks of side effects in a table in a decision aid or in a relatively simple insert located on a prescription drug bottle and to determine which side effect is most likely. With at least a Basic level of performance, patients can be expected to anticipate and plan for medication needs, such as determining how soon a prescription must be ordered based on the number of pills left and the number required each day. One NAAL task identified as at the Intermediate level of performance requires patients to understand medication information and infer, based on instructions, how to handle a missed dose, taking into consideration the time since their last meal.

The management of chronic diseases such as diabetes and asthma pose particular challenges, even for those with Proficient quantitative literacy. Diabetics must know how to accurately use and understand the readings from glucose meters, and modify their insulin dosage based on glucose levels, level of activity, and carbohydrate content. The information needed to make these calculations is found in a variety of formats, such as sliding scales and tables that include nutritional information. Diabetic patients need to be able to perform relatively complex calculations correctly, understand numeric information presented in different formats, and recall numeric information and/or keep an accurate record of it. This combination of tasks is likely more difficult than any of the NAAL examples at the Proficient level. As a result, even the most numerate likely find chronic disease management challenging, although they would perform better than those at lower performance levels.

## QUESTION 3: WHAT DO WE KNOW ABOUT HOW PROVIDERS SHOULD COMMUNICATE WITH THOSE WITH LOW NUMERACY SKILLS?

A series of recent papers has reviewed how to present numeric information to maximize informed decision making (e.g., Ancker et al., 2006; Apter et al., 2008; Berkman et al., 2011; Fagerlin and Peters, 2011; Fagerlin et al., 2007a; Hibbard and Peters, 2003; Lipkus, 2007; Lipkus and Hollands, 1999; Peters et al., 2007a). They have come to many of the same conclusions. In this section, we summarize the literature by focusing on five main communication themes that are consistent with the process goals identified in Figure A-1 (especially lowering cognitive effort and highlighting meaning) and that are updated based on more recent results with less numerate patients and consumers.

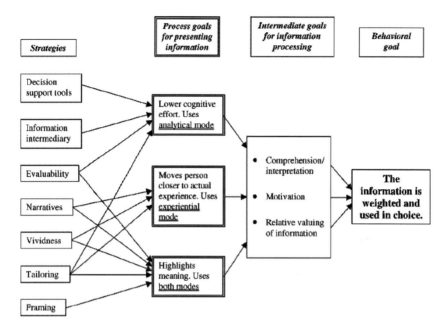

**FIGURE A-1** Data presentation approaches that facilitate informed decision making and the use of information in choice.
SOURCE: Hibbard and Peters, 2003.

Communicators should

- Provide numeric information (as opposed to not providing it);
- Reduce the cognitive effort required from the patient or consumer and require fewer inferences (i.e., do the math for them);
- Provide evaluative meaning, particularly when numeric information is unfamiliar;
- Draw attention to important information; and
- Set up appropriate systems to assist consumers and patients.

Most strategies targeted toward the education-based numeracy skills from Table A-2 can be found in the section focused on reducing cognitive effort. Strategies targeted at the emergent decision-based skills are found in the sections on reducing cognitive effort, providing evaluative meaning, and drawing attention to important information. Table A-6 summarizes recommended strategies for communicating with patients and consumers with low numeracy skills. In the text that follows, we describe the evidence underlying each of these recommendations.

**TABLE A-6** Summary of Recommended Strategies for Communicating with the Less Numerate

| What Communicators Should Do | Specific Strategies |
| --- | --- |
| Provide numeric information (as opposed to not providing it) | Self-explanatory |
| Reduce the cognitive effort required from the patient or consumer and require fewer inferences (i.e., do the math for them) | Provide fewer options<br>Provide less information<br>Present absolute risks, not just relative risks<br>Keep denominators and time spans constant<br>Use numbers consistent with how people use the number line<br>Do the math for them<br>Use appropriate visuals |
| Provide evaluative meaning, particularly when numeric information is unfamiliar | Carefully use evaluative labels and symbols<br>Carefully use frequency versus percentage formats<br>Use other, more imaginable data formats<br>Use emotion to persuade |
| Draw attention to important information | Order information with the most important information first or last<br>Highlight the meaning of only the most important information<br>Use a framework to provide an overview<br>Use fonts that draw attention to important information |
| Set up appropriate systems to assist consumers and patients | Identify communication goals<br>Choose information presentation formats strategically<br>Consider the use of default options and other choice architecture<br>Use computer-aided decision tools<br>Use information intermediaries |

## Provide Numeric Information (as Opposed to Not Providing It)

In consumer domains such as purchases of homes and lottery tickets, numeric information (e.g., mortgage rates and likelihoods of winning) is provided to better inform choices. In health domains, numbers are sometimes provided consistently (e.g., copay amounts in insurance choices), but other times are rarely provided (e.g., likelihoods of benefits and side effects when choosing a medical treatment). Providing numbers (compared to not providing them) even in these latter circumstances has been found to influence patient understanding and willingness to take medications in two ways (Berry, 2006; Lipkus, 2007). First, qualitative labels such as "low chance" or "common" are interpreted differently by different people. To one person, common might mean 50 percent whereas to others it means 25 percent (Berry, 2006). Second, the average person tends to overestimate risk likelihood when provided with only non-numeric information (e.g., risk labels such as "common," "rare") compared to when they are provided numeric information (Berry et al., 2002, 2003a,b). Of course, providing numeric information can be problematic, particularly in less numerate populations. As a result, policy makers and others have questioned whether less numerate populations can "handle" numeric information (Schwartz, 2011). Results of a recent study, however, did not support this view (Peters et al., in review). Both more and less numerate respondents were less likely to overestimate risks and were more willing to take the prescribed medication when provided numeric information about medication side effects as opposed to providing only non-numeric information. Although less numerate individuals have more difficulty with numeric information than do the more numerate, they nonetheless benefitted from its provision at least in the context of medication side effects.

The fact that less numerate individuals do have more problems with numeric information, however, emphasizes the need to understand how to provide comprehensible and usable numeric information to them.

## Reduce the Cognitive Effort Required from the Patient or Consumer and Require Fewer Inferences from Them (i.e., Do the Math for Them)

### Provide Fewer Options

A breast cancer communication tool called "Adjuvant Online!" (http://www.adjuvantonline.com) was designed to help oncologists communicate the benefits for patients receiving hormonal therapy and chemotherapy (Ravdin et al., 2001). Typically, patients are presented with the risks of no additional treatment, each treatment alone, or both hormonal therapy and chemotherapy. However, for most women, only two choices are appropriate. Zikmund-Fisher and colleagues (2008) tested the impact of providing only those two choices and found that, when fewer options were presented, knowledge increased significantly. Medical and other health experts should identify more and less critical elements of a decision (e.g., dominated options that are worse than other available options on every important dimension) so that information providers can delete them from the consideration set or strategically choose how to present them.

Although having more choice options can have advantages, recent research has pointed toward the notion of a "paradox" or "tyranny" of choice. For example, psychological research has demonstrated that having more options can lead to worse choices and lower satisfaction (Hanoch et al., 2009; Schwartz, 2005). In particular, researchers have suggested that an overabundance of choice can lead to information overload (Huffman and Kahn, 1998; Reutskaja and Hogarth, 2009; Scammon, 1977), decreased motivation, an inability to choose (Dhar, 1997; Iyengar and Lepper, 2000; Iyengar et al., 2004), decision-related anxiety (Garbarino and Edell, 1997), and outcome dissatisfaction and regret (Botti and McGill, 2006; Schwartz, 2000, 2004). Schwartz et al. (2002) further found that the combination of large choice sets and a desire to choose the best were related to more regret, reduced happiness, and less overall choice satisfaction. The notion of providing fewer options may be particularly relevant to health plan selection. Numeracy effects have not been studied to the best of our knowledge, but it seems likely that providing fewer options would be especially helpful to the less numerate.

## Provide Less Information

Information is provided to respect consumer and patient autonomy and to help them make better informed decisions. Cognitive drawbacks exist, however, to providing more information. Peters and colleagues (2007a) tested whether providing lay decision makers with less information, rather than more, could result in the best outcomes. The results indicated that providing less information in hospital quality reports (non-quality-of-care information, e.g., the number of general care beds was removed) resulted in better decision making through improved comprehension and higher quality choices, particularly among participants with lower numeracy skills. Health information providers are faced with a challenge to communicate important content to patients and consumers (e.g., through patient portals and mobile apps) and, simultaneously, not communicate too much content as the presence of extraneous information appears to confuse those who are less numerate (see also Kaminski and Sloutsky, 2013).

## Present Absolute Risks, Not Just Relative Risks

When treatment information is presented in a relative risk format (e.g., using hormone replacement therapy doubles the risk of breast cancer), their risks seem larger and treatments are viewed less favorably than when the same information is presented using an absolute risk format (Baron, 1997; Forrow et al., 1992; Malenka et al., 1993). This is as true for the lay public as it is for medical students (Chao et al., 2003). Although not studied with respect to numeracy, it is quite likely that effects would be as big or bigger among the less numerate. Other relative risk examples are ambiguous ("Treatment X has a 5 percent greater risk than Y"). If treatment Y has an absolute risk of 20 percent, 5 percent more risk means that X has a risk of either 21 percent or 25 percent. Providing absolute risk numbers disambiguates the situation and reduces cognitive effort and potential confusion by doing the math for the patient.

## Keep Denominators and Time Spans Constant

Patients experience greater difficulty comparing across treatments when different denominators are used (Fagerlin and Peters, 2011). A single denominator should be chosen for comparisons (e.g., 1 in 10,000 and 400 in 10,000 rather than 1 in 10,000 and 4 in 100). In addition, whole numbers (e.g., 1 in 10,000) are better understood than fractions and decimals (0.01 in 100). Similar advice exists for time spans. To facilitate comparisons, use the same time frame when presenting risks and benefits (e.g., provide annual costs for all health plans rather than monthly costs for some and annual costs for others).

## Use Numbers in a Direction Consistent with People's Expectations

Peters and colleagues (2007a) found that less numerate consumers, in particular, understood more when provided information requiring less cognitive effort. They presented hospital quality-of-care information either in a format in which a higher number meant better (the number of registered nurses per 100 patients) or in the more usual format where a lower number meant better (the number of patients per registered nurse). Putting the numbers in a direction consistent with people's expectations (i.e., usually higher numbers mean something "better" than lower numbers) facilitated comprehension and helped respondents make better choices. Results were even stronger among the less numerate than among the highly numerate. This concept applies equally to other information formats common in medicine. For example, when explaining risks associated with treatment, some information providers use the Number Needed to Treat (NNT). If considering the benefits of chemotherapy, for example, NNT is the number of women needed to take chemoprevention to prevent cancer in one of them; here, larger numbers mean a less effective treatment. NNT is a difficult format for people to understand and it should not be used with laypeople (and arguably not with physicians either who can also be innumerate) (Anderson et al., 2011; Sheridan and Pignone, 2002).

## Do the Math for Them

When evaluating healthy behaviors such as taking medication, eating better, or exercising more, consumers and patients are often told about risks over one time period and they are expected to extrapolate to other time periods. For example, Nina might be informed of the annual risk of taking birth control pills, but she intends to take them for many years, say 10. Understanding this 10-year risk requires a level of numeracy that most people do not have. In one study, for example, well-educated participants were asked a problem that required a similar mathematical solution: "Imagine that, when the Columbus Clippers and the Eugene Emeralds minor league baseball teams have played each other, the Columbus Clippers won only 10 percent of the time. If the teams have a four-game series, by your calculations, what are the chances that the Clippers will win at least once?" (Correct answer: 34 percent) (Peters et al., 2012). Only 1 percent of their college student sample answered this question correctly. Similar cumulative-risk comprehension issues exist in the long-term, false-positive rates from annual cancer screenings in some groups (Gigerenzer, 2002; Sakr et al., 1996; USPSTF, 2011; Welch et al., 2011). Providing estimates for risks over longer time periods by doing the math for consumers would go a long way toward helping them understand the cumulative implications of their choices.

*Use Appropriate Visuals*

Presenting event rates with visual aids such as pictographs (also called icon arrays), bar charts, or flow diagrams may aid accurate understanding of numeric information such as probabilities. This appears particularly true in less numerate populations. Visual displays have been shown to reduce several biases, including denominator neglect (Garcia-Retamero et al., 2010), framing effects (Garcia-Retamero and Cokely, 2011), and the use of anecdotes over more reliable statistical information (Fagerlin et al., 2005a). Icon arrays, in particular, have been tested extensively in recent health communication research, and some nuances to their use have arisen. For example, the icons should be arranged in blocks (e.g., of those with versus without the disease) rather than being scattered randomly (although scattering them randomly can facilitate the perception of randomness, e.g., who gets a disease). Numerator size may also be an important factor when presenting the changes in numeric outcomes for events out of 1,000 among adults with lower education and literacy (McCaffery et al., 2012). Where the outcome is less than 100/1,000, icon arrays were better understood and processed more quickly than bar charts, particularly if the difference between event rates was small. However, for more common outcomes (greater than 100/1,000), bar charts were better, possibly because the icon arrangement was more complicated. In addition, the role of shading in processing the part-to-whole relationship of icon arrays is still not well understood. Most importantly, usually single icon arrays have been tested, and little is known about the effects of icon arrays in those health situations that would likely require integration across multiple arrays (e.g., displaying the 10 possible adverse effects of a prescribed medication). It seems probable that the complexity of multiple icon arrays would disadvantage the less numerate in particular.

Finally, some graphs appeared better suited for particular tasks (e.g., line graphs for trends over time, bar graphs for comparison across groups) (Lipkus, 2007; Lipkus and Hollands, 1999). One final note: Just because consumers or patients prefer some graphs does not necessarily mean they will understand them better than nonpreferred graphs. For an excellent systematic review of the use of graphs in health communication (that did not focus on numeracy, however), see Ancker et al. (2006).

### Provide Evaluative Meaning or Highlight Meaning

Some of the approaches recommended above lower cognitive effort by providing cues to transform the information to an evaluative good/bad scale (Hsee, 1996, 1998). Instead of having to think hard about how to evaluate the goodness or badness of information about an option, an evaluable display reduces the analytical effort required by providing these evaluations in a simpler form. It also may motivate further information processing and behaviors (Peters et al., 2009). The concept of evaluability is simple but profound. Information varies in the degree to which it conveys evaluative meaning. Particularly in unfamiliar domains, we may not know what a measure means (e.g., a measure of quality of care, expressed by the percentage of people satisfied with their care). Research on evaluability demonstrates that even if we understand the numbers used (e.g., a medication that has a 2 percent elevated risk of stroke) at some fundamental level, we may not have an emotional or affective understanding of it (e.g., we do not know how bad this elevated risk is). When information lacks emotional meaning, it lacks evaluability and is not weighted properly in decision making (Slovic et al., 2002). We can determine meaning through considerable effort in comparing and contrasting available information; this is especially true for the highly numerate (Peters et al., 2006a). However, it appears that consumers do not always go to this extra effort and may rely instead on information that is a priori more evaluable. In health contexts, for example, money may be one of the variables that is most evaluable and easily understood; other important variables such as quality-of-care measures are less evaluable and, thus, are less weighted in choice despite their importance to the long-term quality of our health care system. As we will review, however, information evaluability can be improved in a variety of ways. By improving evaluability, we can lower the effort required of the analytical system and highlight the meaning of the information at the same time.

Altering the evaluability of information means that we can help consumers transform data into meaningful information and, by so doing, affect the degree to which the information is actually used in choice (Hibbard et al., 2002). These evaluability changes make all of the information about a choice available in a simple good/bad form (so that consumers can compare apples to apples). This simpler information then influences the interpretation and comprehension of information about the choice attributes. By providing information in an explicitly evaluative form, it can be used more easily to evaluate the overall goodness or badness of any one option. Experimental findings indicate that evaluable displays of comparative data influence the degree to which information such as quality of care is actually weighted and used in choice.

## Carefully Use Evaluative Labels and Symbols

People making decisions can be quite poor at using numeric information in making decisions. Interpreting the meaning of numeric information (e.g., telling patients how good or bad a 9 percent risk is) can have a robust influence in health judgments and choices across diverse adult populations (Peters et al., 2009). In one series of studies, providing evaluative labels (poor, fair, good, and excellent) with numeric quality-of-care information resulted in its greater use in judgments and less reliance on an irrelevant affective state among the less numerate. Follow-up studies in this paper demonstrated that consumers given evaluative labels processed the numeric information (and did not ignore it due to the presence of labels). Instead, the evaluative labels appeared to increase the relative accessibility of valenced feelings about the choice options over valenced thoughts about the same options. In another study, evaluative labels for test results (that a test came back "positive" or "abnormal") induced larger changes to risk perceptions and behavioral intentions than did numeric results alone (Zikmund-Fisher et al., 2007). The normative appropriateness of changes in this latter study were unclear, however, thus highlighting that evaluative labels should be applied with great care.

## Carefully Use Frequency Versus Percentage Formats

The choice between frequencies and percentages can affect people's perceptions of provided information, especially risk information (Slovic et al., 2000). For instance, Peters and colleagues asked participants to imagine they had severe headaches and that a medicine existed that could decrease headache frequency (Peters et al., 2011). Participants read about a possible side effect of the drug in a percentage format (10 percent of patients get a blistering rash) or in a frequency format (10 patients out of 100 get a blistering rash). Less numerate participants (but not the highly numerate) perceived the medicine as less risky when side effect information was presented using percentages rather than frequencies. Peters et al. interpreted their results as being due to the frequency formats eliciting greater emotional imagery compared to percentage formats (thought to be perceived as relatively abstract and meaningless). Because information providers have to choose some format to provide likelihood information (and no format is neutral), they should think carefully about whether they would recommend taking a medication that has a possible side effect (in which case, they should use a percentage format in conveying possible risks) or they think the patient should seriously consider the side effect (they might use a frequency format instead). The choice of format will make little difference to the highly numerate, but will matter to the less numerate (see also Dieckmann et al., 2009; Peters et al., 2006b).

*Use Other More Imaginable Data Formats*

Just as data presented in a frequentistic format may be easier (and more emotional) to imagine than presented in a probabilistic format, changes in life expectancy appear easier to imagine than changes in disease risk. Galesic and Garcia-Retamero (2011) found that, when information about consequences of risky behaviors was presented as months of life lost or gained, recall was better than when it was presented in terms of risks of a disease. The effect held for both short-term and longer-term memory for the information and for individuals higher and lower in numeracy. The improved recall seemed to be due to better imaginability of changes in life expectancy. These results are consistent with recent research demonstrating an effect of displaying the minutes of brisk walking needed to burn calories for menu items (as opposed to having only calorie counts) on how many calories were ordered and consumed (James et al., 2013).

*Use Emotion to Persuade*

Diverse studies have demonstrated that affective reactions are powerful sources of information when deriving perceptions of risk (Loewenstein et al., 2001; Slovic et al., 2004). Emotional manipulations can influence risk evaluations (Loewenstein et al., 2001; Slovic et al., 2004) and increase thoughts about behavioral change (Diefenbach et al., 1999; Romer and Jamieson, 2001). Tobacco, for example, is the leading cause of preventable death worldwide, killing one person every 6 seconds (CDC, 2012; WHO, 2012). To combat this epidemic, some countries have implemented health warnings on the front and back of cigarette packages that include basic statements of health risks (e.g., "smoking kills") and large graphic images illustrating the risks. In contrast to basic text-only warnings, which are forgettable and ineffective (Bansal-Travers et al., 2011; Borland et al., 2009;

Hammond et al., 2007; Moodie et al., 2009), graphic pictorial warnings create negative affect toward smoking (Peters et al., 2007c) and encourage smokers with those reactions to think about quitting (Hammond, 2011; White et al., 2008). It is thought that the graphic labels may have greater effects among less educated (including less numerate) populations. Health care providers should consider the use of emotion such as with graphic verbal or visual representations in situations where persuasion is an acceptable tool.

## Draw Attention to Important Information

### Order Information So That the Most Important Information Is First or Last

Ordering information can help consumers by reducing the cognitive effort required to locate and understand the goodness or badness of information and by drawing attention to important information. Hibbard et al. (2002), for example, found that ordering health plans by performance within premium cost strata resulted in more choices of higher performing plans compared with presenting the information unordered. It is not clear from the literature whether ordering might have a differential effect based on consumer numeracy level, but it is likely that the effect is larger among the less numerate, who generally have more difficulty understanding the meaning of numeric information.

### Highlight the Meaning of Only the Most Important Information

In Peters et al. (2007a), making only a more important quality measure easier to evaluate through the use of evaluative symbols such as those used by *Consumer Reports* (rather than making all indicators easier to evaluate) led to more choices of higher quality hospitals. These results were particularly strong among the less numerate. When the meaning of nonessential information is highlighted (along with more important information being highlighted), it may actually worsen health choices among those with lower numeracy.

### Use a Framework to Provide an Overview

Greene et al. (2008) examined consumer understanding and use of information when making a choice between a more familiar type of health plan and a less familiar one. They found that less numerate consumers understood less of the information provided about the new type of health plan at the same time as they were substantially more likely to choose it.

Providing an overarching framework to explain and highlight the differences between the two types of health plans boosted comprehension of items related to the framework message. However, it reduced comprehension of items not related to the framework, particularly among the less numerate. The study highlighted the difficulty that many consumers, and especially the less numerate, have in understanding comparative plan information and in making informed health care choices similar to what will be provided as a result of the ACA. Providing a framework can help, but information providers will need to take care that all important information is mentioned in the framework (with the more detailed information following the framework) to ensure comprehension among the less numerate.

*Use Fonts That Draw Attention to Important Information*

One reason that health information may not be used is because consumers never attended to it in the first place. With numeric information, this may be particularly true for less numerate consumers (see review of attention effects in the section on emergent decision-based numeracy skills). Methods can be used, however, to explicitly draw attention to numeric information in these cases. Stimuli that are perceptually salient draw attention (Parkhurst et al., 2002) and tend to have greater influence on choice (Bettman et al., 1998). For example, in a men's clothing store, a red tie placed in a display of neutrally colored ties may capture attention and be chosen more often than the same red tie in a display of vibrant colors.

The visual salience of health information can be manipulated in a variety of ways, including through larger or bold fonts. In an unpublished dissertation, for example, Sagara (2009) found that participants were more sensitive to different levels of numeric information when the numbers were printed in a font that contrasted more with other information provided. In particular, numeric product information that was italicized and printed in grey (in contrast with the regular black font of the surrounding information) appeared to increase the salience of the numeric information, and to result in a greater impact of the numbers on participants' product judgments. In two studies in an unpublished master's thesis, Meilleur (2012) varied the risks associated with a vaccination and the font size in which the risks were printed to increase salience and draw attention to the risks. Meilleur found that increasing the font size of the numeric risk information drew participants' attention toward it, increased their sensitivity to risk, and altered vaccination decisions.

## Set Up Appropriate Systems

### Identify the Goals of the Communication

To communicate effectively, communicators (whether health care providers or insurance providers) need to identify the goal or goals of a communication and what information the decision maker needs to receive. Without this identification of what matters and to whom, communication efforts will be inadequate. For the previously uninsured population, low numeracy is likely to be an issue. Communication efforts (how to present information) should address this issue in an evidence-based manner. For each type of decision the previously uninsured population will need to make, effective communication will depend in part on identifying information that is more and less important and identifying options that are dominated and dominant. Doing so will allow communicators to take some of the recommended steps to reduce cognitive effort, highlight evaluative meaning, and draw attention to important information in ways that facilitate appropriate comprehension and use of numeric information.

### Information Presentation Formats

Communication should be viewed as a strategic process that begins with identifying which information the patient or consumer should know and use or wants to know and use. Then information presentation should proceed in an evidence-based manner to best reach the identified communication goals. One of the most important points is that communications should be tested prior to their use and in appropriate populations (e.g., in a less numerate population if that is the ultimate target for the communication).

### Default Options and Other Choice Architecture

If a health provider wants to promote behavior change (as opposed to simply informing a patient or consumer), the notion of choice architecture offers alternative approaches to promoting better health decisions. Choice architecture is a term coined by Thaler and Sunstein (2008) that reflects the fact that many ways exist to present a choice to decision makers, and that what is chosen often depends on how the choice is presented. Although few of these tools have been examined with respect to individual differences such as numeracy, they hold some promise. Johnson et al. (2012) provide a brief review that identifies, describes, and categorizes some of the many tools that could be tested within health environments.

One of the primary tools tested thus far is the use of default options.

Defaults are choice options that are chosen a priori by policy makers and that are applied to individuals who do not take active steps to change away from them (Brown and Krishna, 2004). The default is "chosen" if the consumer does nothing. These are already in wide use; consider, for example, a physician who has a recommended treatment. She usually just writes out the appropriate prescription at that point, although the patient could continue to discuss alternative treatments. Defaults have been shown to have strong effects on choices concerning investments (Cronqvist and Thaler, 2004; Madrian and Shea, 2001), insurance (Johnson et al., 2003), and organ donation (Johnson and Goldstein, 2003). They appeal to a wide audience in their ability to guide choice while preserving freedom of choice. In another example, providing calorie information has not consistently improved individuals' food choices. However, providing healthful default options on a menu has significantly increased choices of lower calorie foods (Wisdom et al., 2010). Greater use of defaults may be particularly useful in health insurance selection to encourage enrollment and, if defaults are carefully selected, result in consumers who are more likely to be satisfied with their choice.

### Computer-Aided Decision Tools

Health care and related providers do not need to be the sole communicators with the ACA population. Many of the same strategies (e.g., reducing cognitive burden and highlighting meaning) can be accomplished through the use of carefully designed, computer-aided decision tools. Use of such tools can structure and simplify the decision process at the same time as important factors and trade-offs are highlighted for consideration. Calculators (e.g., for health plan costs for those needing a lot of health care because of chronic disease or those expecting few health care costs) can be built into such tools or can be provided as stand-alone tools. Such strategies may be quite important given the small proportion of the ACA population expected to have Proficient levels of quantitative literacy and to be able to perform such calculations (see Table A-3).

### Intermediary

Individuals sometimes require greater assistance, particularly individuals with less computer experience, lower numeracy, and other limitations with respect to health literacy. An information intermediary can perform a similar, but more personalized, function to computer-aided decision tools.

## CONCLUSIONS

The expected influx of previously uninsured individuals into our nation's health care system will present a variety of challenges, including the challenges of communicating with less numerate individuals who have limited knowledge and abilities to navigate this unfamiliar and often numeric world. This population will vary considerably in education-based numeracy skills (from basic arithmetic to understanding cumulative risk) and emergent decision-based numeracy skills (from seeking out numeric information to deriving affective meaning from it). Providers have an opportunity in the coming months and years to better understand who these people are (in terms of their abilities) and to apply the science of communication to help these patients and consumers make informed decisions and maximize their health and well-being given new ACA benefits.

## REFERENCES

Abaluck, J., and J. Gruber. 2011. Choice inconsistencies among the elderly: Evidence from Plan Choice in the Medicare Part D program. *American Economic Review* 101(4):1180-1210.

Ancker, J. S., and D. R. Kaufman. 2007. Rethinking health numeracy: A multidisciplinary literature review. *Journal of the American Medical Informatics Association* 14(6):713-721.

Ancker, J. S., Y. Senathirajah, R. Kukafka, and J. B. Starren. 2006. Design features of graphs in health risk communication: A systematic review. *Journal of the American Medical Informatics Association* 13:608-618.

Anderson, B. L., N. A. Obrecht, G. B. Chapman, D. A. Driscoll, and J. Schulkin. 2011. Physicians' communication of Down syndrome screening test results: The influence of physician numeracy. *Genetics in Medicine* 13:744-749.

Apter, A. J., J. Cheng, D. Small, I. M. Bennett, C. Albert, D. G. Fein, M. George, and S. Van Horne. 2006. Asthma numeracy skill and health literacy. *Journal of Asthma* 43:705-710.

Apter, A. J., M. K. Paasche-Orlow, J. T. Remillard, I. M. Bennett, E. P. Ben-Joseph, R. M. Batista, J. Hyde, and R. E. Rudd. 2008. Numeracy and communication with patients: They are counting on us. *Journal of General Internal Medicine* 23(12):2117-2124.

Bansal-Travers, M., D. Hammond, P. Smith, and M. Cummings. 2011. The impact of cigarette pack design, descriptors, and warning labels on risk perception in the U.S. *American Journal of Preventative Medicine* 40(6):674-682.

Baron, J. 1997. Confusion of relative and absolute risk in valuation. *Journal of Risk and Uncertainty* 14:301-309.

Bateman, I., S. Dent, E. Peters, P. Slovic, and C. Starmer. 2007. The affect heuristic and the attractiveness of simple gambles. *Journal of Behavioral Decision Making* 20:365-380.

Ben-Joseph, E. P., S. A. Dowshen, and N. Izenberg. 2009. Do parents understand growth charts? A national, Internet-based survey. *Pediatrics* 124:1100-1109.

Berkman, N. D., S. L. Sheridan, K. E. Donahue, D. J. Halpern, A. Viera, K. Crotty, A. Holland, M. Brasure, K. N. Lohr, E. Harden, E. Tant, I. Wallace, and M. Viswanathan. 2011. *Health literacy interventions and outcomes: An updated systematic review.* Evidence Report/Technology Assessment No. 199. (Prepared by RTI International–University of North Carolina Evidence-based Practice Center under contract No. 290-2007-10056-I.) AHRQ Pub. No. 11-E006. Rockville, MD: Agency for Healthcare Research and Quality.

Berry, D. C. 2006. Informing people about the risks and benefits of medicines: Implications for the safe and effective use of medicinal products. *Current Drug Safety* 1:121-126.

Berry, D. C., P. R. Knapp, and D. K. Raynor. 2002. Provision of information about drug side effects to patients. *Lancet* 359:853-854.

Berry, D. C., P. Knapp, and D. K. Raynor. 2003a. Communicating risk of medication side effects: An empirical evaluation of EU recommended terminology. *Psychology, Health & Medicine* 8(3):251-263.

Berry, D. C., D. K. Raynor, P. Knapp, and E. Bersellini. 2003b. Patients' understanding of risk associated with medication use: Impact of European Commission Guidelines and other risk scales. *Drug Society* 26(1):1-11.

Bettman, J. R., M. F. Luce, and J. W. Payne. 1998. Constructive consumer choice processes. *Journal of Consumer Research* 25(3):187-217.

Borland, R., N. Wilson, G. T. Fong, D. Hammond, K. M. Cummings, H. H. Yong, W. Hosking, G. Hastings, J. Thrasher, and A. McNeill. 2009. Impact of graphic and text warnings on cigarette packs: Findings from four countries over five years. *Tobacco Control* 18(5):358-364.

Botti, S., and A. L. McGill. 2006. When choosing is not deciding: The effect of perceived responsibility on satisfaction. *Journal of Consumer Research* 33:211-219.

Brown, C., and A. Krishna. 2004. The skeptical shopper: A metacognitive account for the effects of default options on choice. *Journal of Consumer Research* 31(3):529-539.

CDC (Centers for Disease Control and Prevention). 2012. *Smoking & tobacco use: Fast facts*. http://www.cdc.gov/tobacco/data_statistics/fact_sheets/fast_facts (accessed June 25, 2014).

Chao, C., J. L. Studts, T. Abell, T. Hadley, L. Roetzer, S. Dineen, D. Lorenz, A.Y. Agha, and K. M. McMasters. 2003. Adjuvant chemotherapy for breast cancer: How presentation of recurrence risk influences decision-making. *Journal of Clinical Oncology* 21:4299-4305.

CMS (Centers for Medicare & Medicaid Services). 2013. *Medicare provider charge data*. https://www.cms.gov/Research-Statistics-Data-and-Systems/Statistics-Trends-and-Reports/Medicare-Provider-Charge-Data/index.html (accessed June 25, 2014).

Cokely, E. T., M. Galesic, E. Schulz, S. Ghazal, and R. Garcia-Retamero. 2012. Measuring risk literacy: The Berlin Numeracy Test. *Judgment and Decision Making* 7(1):25-47.

Cronqvist, H., and R. H. Thaler. 2004. Design choices in privatized social-security systems: Learning from the Swedish experience. *American Economic Review* 94(2):424-428.

Damasio, A. R. 1994. *Descartes' error: Emotion, reason, and the human brain*. New York: Avon.

Day, R., and P. Nadash. 2012. New state insurance exchanges should follow the example of Massachusetts by simplifying choices among health plans. *Health Affairs* 31(5):982-989.

Denes-Raj, V., and S. Epstein. 1994. Conflict between intuitive and rational processing: When people behave against their better judgment. *Journal of Personality and Social Psychology* 66:819-829.

Dhar, R. 1997. Consumer preference for a no-choice option. *Journal of Consumer Research* 24:215-231.

Dieckmann, N. F., P. Slovic, and E. M. Peters. 2009. The use of narrative evidence and explicit likelihood by decisionmakers varying in numeracy. *Risk Analysis* 29(10):1473-1488.

Diefenbach, M. A., S. M. Miller, and M. Daly. 1999. Specific worry about breast cancer predicts mammography use in women at risk for breast and ovarian cancer. *Health Psychology* 18:532-536.

Epstein, S. 1994. Integration of the cognitive and the psychodynamic unconscious. *American Psychologist* 49:709-724.

Estrada, C. A., M. Martin-Hryniewicz, B. T. Peek, C. Collins, and J. C. Byrd. 2004. Literacy and numeracy skills and anticoagulation control. *American Journal of the Medical Sciences* 328(2):88-93.

Fagerlin, A., and E. Peters. 2011. Quantitative information. In *Evidence-based communication of risk and benefits: A user's guide*, edited by B. Fischhoff, N. Brewer, and J. Downs. Silver Spring, MD: Food and Drug Administration. Pp. 53-64.

Fagerlin, A., C. Wang, and P. A. Ubel. 2005a. Reducing the influence of anecdotal reasoning on people's health care decisions: Is a picture worth a thousand statistics? *Medical Decision Making* 25(4):398-405.

Fagerlin, A., B. J. Zikmund-Fisher, and P. A. Ubel. 2005b. How making a risk estimate can change the feel of that risk: Shifting attitudes toward breast cancer risk in a general public survey. *Patient Education and Counseling* 57:294-299.

Fagerlin, A., P. A. Ubel, D. M. Smith, and B. J. Zikmund-Fisher. 2007a. Making numbers matter: Present and future research in risk communication. *American Journal of Health Behavior* 31:47-56.

Fagerlin, A., B. J. Zikmund-Fisher, P. A. Ubel, A. Jankovic, H. A. Derry, and D. M. Smith. 2007b. Measuring numeracy without a math test: Development of the Subjective Numeracy Scale. *Medical Decision Making* 27(5):672-680.

Finucane, M. L., A. Alhakami, P. Slovic, and S. M. Johnson. 2000. The affect heuristic in judgments of risks and benefits. *Journal of Behavioral Decision Making* 13:1-17.

Forrow, L., W. C. Taylor, and R. M. Arnold. 1992. Absolutely relative: How research results are summarized can affect treatment decisions. *American Journal of Medicine* 92:121-124.

Galesic, M., and R. Garcia-Retamero. 2010. Statistical numeracy for health: A cross-cultural comparison with probabilistic national samples. *Archives of Internal Medicine* 170(5):462-468.

Galesic, M., and R. Garcia-Retamero. 2011. Communicating consequences of risky behaviors: Life expectancy versus risk of disease. *Patient Education and Counseling* 82:30-35.

Garbarino, E. C., and J. A. Edell. 1997. Cognitive effort, affect, and choice. *Journal of Consumer Research* 24:147-158.

Garcia-Retamero, R., and E. T. Cokely. 2011. Effective communication of risks to young adults: Using message framing and visual aids to increase condom use and STD screening. *Journal of Experimental Psychology: Applied* 17:270-287.

Garcia-Retamero, R., M. Galesic, and G. Gigerenzer. 2010. Do icon arrays help reduce denominator neglect? *Medical Decision Making* 30:672-684.

Gigerenzer, G. 2002. *Calculated risks: How to know when numbers deceive you.* New York: Simon & Schuster.

Greene, J., E. Peters, C. K. Mertz, and J. H. Hibbard. 2008. Comprehension and choice of a consumer-directed health plan: An experimental study. *American Journal of Managed Care* 14(6):369-376.

Hammond, D. 2011. Health warnings on tobacco packages: A review. *Tobacco Control* 20:327-337.

Hammond, D., F. Wiebel, L. T. Kozlowski, R. Borland, K. M. Cummings, R. J. O'Connor, A. McNeill, G. N. Connolly, D. Arnott, and G. T. Fong. 2007. Revising the machine smoking regime for cigarette emissions: Implications for tobacco control policy. *Tobacco Control* 16(1):8-14.

Hanoch, Y., T. Rice, J. Cummings, and S. Wood. 2009. How much choice is too much? The case of the Medicare prescription drug benefit. *Health Services Research* 44(4):1157-1168.

Hibbard, J. H., and E. Peters. 2003. Supporting informed consumer health care choices: Data presentation approaches that facilitate the use of information in choice. *Annual Review of Public Health* 24:413-433.

Hibbard, J. H., P. Slovic, E. M. Peters, M. Finucane, and M. Tusler. 2001. Is the informed-choice approach appropriate for Medicare beneficiaries? *Health Affairs* 20(3):199-203.

Hibbard, J. H., P. Slovic, E. Peters, and M. L. Finucane. 2002. Strategies for reporting health plan performance information to consumers: Evidence from controlled studies. *Health Services Research* 37(2):291-313.

Hibbard, J. H., E. Mahoney, R. Stock, and M. Tusler. 2007a. Do increases in patient activation result in improved self-management behaviors? *Health Services Research* 42(4): 1443-1463.

Hibbard, J. H., E. Peters, A. Dixon, and M. Tusler. 2007b. Consumer competencies and the use of comparative quality information: It isn't just about literacy. *Medical Care Research & Review* 64(4):379-394.

Hsee, C. K. 1996. The evaluability hypothesis: An explanation for preference reversals between joint and separate evaluations of alternatives. *Organizational Behavior and Human Decision Processes* 67:247-257.

Hsee, C. K. 1998. Less is better: When low-value options are valued more highly than high-value options. *Journal of Behavioral Decision Making* 11:107-121.

Huffman, C., and B. E. Kahn. 1998. Variety for sale: Mass customization or mass confusion? *Journal of Retailing* 74:491-513.

Huizinga, M. M., T. A. Elasy, K. A. Wallston, K. Cavanaugh, D. Davis, R. P. Gregory, L. S. Fuchs, R. Malone, A. Cherrington, D. A. DeWalt, J. Buse, M. Pignone, and R. L. Rothman. 2008. Development and validation of the Diabetes Numeracy Test (DNT). *BMC Health Services Research* 8:96.

Iyengar, S. S., and M. R. Lepper. 2000. When choice is demotivating: Can one desire too much of a good thing? *Journal of Personality and Social Psychology* 79:995-1006.

Iyengar, S. S., G. Huberman, and W. Jiang. 2004. How much choice is too much: Determinants of individual contributions in 401K retirement plans. In *Pension design and structure: New lessons from behavioral finance*, edited by O. S. Mitchell and S. Utkus. Oxford, England: Oxford University Press. Pp. 83-95.

James, A., B. Adams-Huet, K. Crisp, J. Mitchell, L. Dart, M. Turner, M. Kasper, J. Bowman, S. Joeckel, N. Toomey, H. Heefner, E. Blasco, and M. Shah. 2013. The effect of menu labels, displaying minutes of brisk walking needed to burn food calories, on calories ordered and consumed in young adults. *Journal of the Federation of American Societies for Experimental Biology* 27:367.2.

Johnson, E. J., and D. G. Goldstein. 2003. Do defaults save lives? *Science* 302:1338-1339.

Johnson, E. J., S. B. Shu, B. G. C. Dellaert, C. Fox, D. G. Goldstein, G. Häubl, R. P. Larrick, J. W. Payne, E. Peters, D. Schkade, B. Wansink, and E. U. Weber. 2012. Beyond nudges: Tools of a choice architecture. *Marketing Letters* 23:487-504.

Johnson, R. W., A. J. Davidoff, and K. Perese. 2003. Health insurance costs and early retirement decisions. *Industrial and Labor Relations Review* 56(4):716-729.

Kahneman, D. 2003. A perspective on judgment and choice: Mapping bounded rationality. *American Psychologist* 58(9):697-720.

Kaminski, J. A., and V. M. Sloutsky. 2013. Extraneous perceptual information interferes with children's acquisition of mathematical knowledge. *Journal of Educational Psychology* 105(2):351-363.

Keller, C. 2011. Using a familiar risk comparison within a risk ladder to improve risk understanding by low numerates: A study of visual attention. *Risk Analysis* 31:1043-1054.

Kutner, M., E. Greenberg, Y. Jin, B. Boyle, Y. Hsu, and E. Dunleavy. 2007. Literacy in everyday life: Results from the 2003 National Assessment of Adult Literacy (NAAL). National Center for Education Statistics. Institute of Education Sciences. http://nces.ed.gov/naal (accessed June 25, 2014).

Lipkus, I. M. 2007. Numeric, verbal, and visual formats of conveying health risks: Suggested best practices and future recommendations. *Medical Decision Making* 27:696-713.

Lipkus, I. M., and J. G. Hollands. 1999. The visual communication of risk. *Journal of the National Cancer Institute Monographs* 9(25):149-163.

Lipkus, I. M., and E. Peters. 2009. Understanding the role of numeracy in health: Proposed theoretical framework and practical insights. *Health Education and Behavior* 36(6):1065-1081.

Lipkus, I. M., G. Samsa, and B. K. Rimer. 2001. General performance on a numeracy scale among highly educated samples. *Medical Decision Making* 21:37-44.

Lipkus, I. M., E. Peters, G. Kimmick, V. Liotcheva, and P. Marcom. 2010. Breast cancer patients' treatment expectations after exposure to the decision aid program Adjuvant Online: The influence of numeracy. *Medical Decision Making* 30:464-473.

Loewenstein, G. F., E. U. Weber, C. K. Hsee, and E. S. Welch. 2001. Risk as feelings. *Psychological Bulletin* 127:267-286.

Madlon-Kay, D. J., and F. S. Mosch. 2000. Liquid medication dosing errors. *Journal of Family Practice* 49(8):741-744.

Madrian, B. C., and D. F. Shea. 2001. The power of suggestion: Inertia in 401(k) participation and savings behavior. *Quarterly Journal of Economics* 116(4):1149-1187.

Malenka, D. J., J. A. Baron, S. Johansen, J. W. Wahrenberger, and J. M. Ross. 1993. The framing effect of relative and absolute risk. *Journal of General Internal Medicine* 8(10): 543-548.

McCaffery, K. J., A. Dixon, A. Hayen, J. Jansen, S. Smith, and J. M. Simpson. 2012. The influence of graphic display format on the interpretations of quantitative risk information among adults with lower education and literacy: A randomized experimental study. *Medical Decision Making* 32(4):532-544.

Meilleur, L. R. 2012. *Manipulating attention to improve health behaviors.* Master's thesis. Ohio State University. Retrieved from OhioLink ETD. Pub. No. OSU1354291552.

Moodie, C., A. M. MacKintosh, and D. Hammond. 2009. Adolescents' response to text-only tobacco health warnings: Results from the 2008 UK Youth Tobacco Policy Survey. *European Journal of Public Health* 20(4):463-469.

Parkhurst, D., K. Law, and E. Niebur. 2002. Modeling the role of salience in the allocation of overt visual attention. *Vision Research* 42:107-123.

Peters, E. 2012. Beyond comprehension: The role of numeracy in judgments and decisions. *Current Directions in Psychological Science* 21(1):31-35.

Peters, E., D. Västfjäll, T. Gärling, and P. Slovic. 2006a. Affect and decision making: A "hot" topic. *Journal of Behavioral Decision Making* 19(2):79-85.

Peters, E., D. Västfjäll, P. Slovic, C. K. Mertz, K. Mazzocco, and S. Dickert. 2006b. Numeracy and decision making. *Psychological Science* 17(5):407-413.

Peters, E., N. Dieckmann, A. Dixon, J. H. Hibbard, and C. K. Mertz. 2007a. Less is more in presenting quality information to consumers. *Medical Care Research & Review* 64(2):169-190.

Peters, E., J. Hibbard, P. Slovic, and N. Dieckmann. 2007b. Numeracy skill and the communication, comprehension, and use of risk-benefit information. *Health Affairs* 26(3):741-748.

Peters, E., D. Romer, P. Slovic, K. H. Jamieson, L. Wharfield, C. K. Mertz, and S. M. Carpenter. 2007c. The impact and acceptability of Canadian-style cigarette warning labels among U.S. smokers and nonsmokers. *Nicotine & Tobacco Research* 9(4):473-481.

Peters, E., N. F. Dieckmann, D. Västfjäll, C. K. Mertz, P. Slovic, and J. H. Hibbard. 2009. Bringing meaning to numbers: The impact of evaluative categories on decisions. *Journal of Experimental Psychology: Applied* 15(3):213-227.

Peters, E., S. Hart, and L. Fraenkel. 2011. Informing patients: The influence of numeracy, framing, and format of side effect information on risk perceptions. *Medical Decision Making* 31(3):432-436.

Peters, E., H. Kunreuther, N. Sagara, P. Slovic, and D. R. Schley. 2012. Protective measures, personal experience, and the affective psychology of time. *Risk Analysis* 32(12):2084-2097.

Peters, E., S. Hart, M. Tusler, and L. Fraenkel. In review. Numbers matter to informed patient choices: The effects of age and numeracy.

Quincy, L. 2012. State insurance exchanges' impact on consumers. In *Facilitating state health exchange communication through the use of health literate practices: Workshop summary*. Washington, DC: The National Academies Press. Pp. 27-47.

Ratzan, S. C., and R. M. Parker. 2000. Introduction. In *National Library of Medicine current bibliographies in medicine: Health literacy*, edited by C. R. Selden, M. Zorn, S. C. Ratzan, and R. M. Parker. Bethesda, MD: National Institutes of Health.

Ravdin, P. M., L. A. Siminoff, G. J. Davis, M. B. Mercer, J. Hewlett, N. Gerson, and H. L. Parker. 2001. Computer program to assist in making decisions about adjuvant therapy for women with early breast cancer. *Journal of Clinical Oncology* 19(4):980-991.

Reutskaja, E., and R. M. Hogarth. 2009. Satisfaction in choice as a function of the number of alternatives: When "goods satiate." *Psychology & Marketing* 26(3):197-203.

Reyna, V. F. 2004. How people make decisions that involve risk: A dual-processes approach. *Current Directions in Psychological Science* 13:60-66.

Reyna, V. F., W. L. Nelson, P. K. Han, and N. F. Dieckmann. 2009. How numeracy influences risk comprehension and medical decision making. *Psychological Bulletin* 135:943-973.

Romer, D., and P. Jamieson. 2001. Do adolescents appreciate the risks of smoking?: Evidence from a national survey. *Journal of Adolescent Health* 29:12-21.

Rosenthal, J. A., X. Lu, and P. Cram. 2013. Availability of consumer prices from US hospitals for a common surgical procedure. *JAMA Internal Medicine* 173(6):427-432.

Sagara, N. 2009. *Consumer understanding and use of numeric information in product claims*. Doctoral dissertation. University of Oregon. Retrieved from ProQuest. Pub. No. AAT 3395194.

Sakr, W. A., D. J. Gringon, G. P. Hass, L. K. Heilbrun, J. E. Pontes, and J. D. Crissman. 1996. Age and racial distribution of prostatic intraepithelial neoplasia. *European Urology* 30(2):138-144.

Scammon, D. L. 1977. Information load and consumers. *Journal of Consumer Research* 4:148-155.

Schwartz, B. 2000. Self-determination: The tyranny of freedom. *American Psychologist* 55: 79-88.

Schwartz, B. 2004. *The paradox of choice*. New York: Harper Collins Publishers.

Schwartz, B. 2005. Choose and lose. *New York Times*, January 5.

Schwartz, B., A. Ward, J. Monterosso, S. Lyubomirsky, K. White, and D. R. Lehman. 2002. Maximizing versus satisficing: Happiness is a matter of choice. *Journal of Personality and Social Psychology* 83(5):1178-1197.

Schwartz, P. H. 2011. Questioning the quantitative imperative: Decision aids, prevention, and the ethics of disclosure. *Hastings Center Report* 41(2):30-39.

Shapira, M. M., C. M. Walker, K. J. Cappaert, P. S. Ganschow, K. E. Fletcher, E. L. McGinley, S. Del Pozo, C. Schauer, S. Tarima, and E. A. Jacobs. 2012. The Numeracy Understanding in Medicine instrument (NUMi): A measure of health numeracy developed using Item Response Theory. *Medical Decision Making* 32:851-865.

Sheridan, S. L., and M. Pignone. 2002. Numeracy and the medical student's ability to interpret data. *Effective Clinical Practice* 5:35-40.

Shiv, B., and A. Fedorikhin. 1999. Heart and mind in conflict: The interplay of affect and cognition in consumer decision making. *Journal of Consumer Research* 26(3):278-292.

Sloman, S. A. 1996. The empirical case for two systems of reasoning. *Psychological Bulletin* 119:3-22.

Slovic, P., J. Monahan, and D. G. MacGregor. 2000. Violence risk assessment and risk communication: The effects of using actual cases, providing instructions, and employing probability versus frequency formats. *Law and Human Behavior* 24:271-296.

Slovic, P., M. Finucane, E. Peters, and D. G. MacGregor. 2002. Rational actors or rational fools: Implications of the affect heuristic for behavioral economics. *Journal of Socio-Economics* 31(4):329-342.

Slovic, P., M. L. Finucane, E. Peters, and D. G. MacGregor. 2004. Risk as analysis and risk as feelings: Some thoughts about affect, reason, risk, and rationality. *Risk Analysis* 24(2): 311-322.

Slovic, P., E. Peters, M. L. Finucane, and D. G. MacGregor. 2005. Affect, risk, and decision making. *Health Psychology* 24:S35-S40.

Stanovich, K. E., and R. F. West. 2002. Individual differences in reasoning: Implications for the rationality debate? In *Heuristics and biases: The psychology of intuitive judgment*, edited by T. Gilovich, D. W. Griffin, and D. Kahneman. New York: Cambridge University Press. Pp. 421-440.

Thaler, R. H., and C. R. Sunstein. 2008. *Nudge: Improving decisions about health, wealth and happiness*. New Haven, CT: Yale University Press.

U.S. Census Bureau. 2009-2011. *Selected characteristics of the uninsured in the United States 2009-2011*. http://factfinder2.census.gov (accessed June 25, 2014).

U.S. Census Bureau. 2012. *Health insurance: Highlights*. http://www.census.gov/hhes/www/hlthins/data/incpovhlth/2011/highlights.html (accessed June 25, 2014).

USPSTF (U.S. Preventive Services Task Force). 2011, October. *Screening for prostate cancer: A review of the evidence for the U.S. Preventive Services Task Force*. http://www.uspreventiveservicestaskforce.org/uspstf/uspsprca.htm (accessed June 25, 2014).

Västfjäll, D., E. Peters, and C. Starmer. In preparation. Numeracy, incidental affect and the construction of prices.

Welch, G., L. Schwartz, and S. Woloshin. 2011. *Overdiagnosed: Making people sick in the pursuit of health*. Boston, MA: Beacon Press.

Weller, J., N. F. Dieckmann, M. Tusler, C. K. Mertz, W. Burns, and E. Peters. 2013. Development and testing of an abbreviated numeracy scale: A Rasch Analysis approach. *Journal of Behavioral Decision Making* 26(2):198-212.

White, V., B. Webster, and M. Wakefield. 2008. Do graphic health warning labels have an impact on adolescents' smoking-related beliefs and behaviours? *Addiction* 103(9):1562-1571.

WHO (World Health Organization). 2012. *Tobacco*. http://www.who.int/mediacentre/factsheets/fs339/en/index.html (accessed June 25, 2014).

Wisdom, J., J. S. Downs, and G. Loewenstein. 2010. Promoting healthy choices: Information versus convenience. *American Economic Journal: Applied Economics* 2:164-178.

Zikmund-Fisher, B. J., A. Fagerlin, K. Keeton, and P. A. Ubel. 2007. Does labeling prenatal screening test results as negative or positive affect a woman's responses? *American Journal of Obstetrics and Gynecology* 197:528.e1-528.e6.

Zikmund-Fisher, B. J., A. Fagerlin, and P. A. Ubel. 2008. Improving understanding of adjuvant therapy options via simpler risk graphics. *Cancer* 113(12):3382-3390.

Zikmund-Fisher, B. J., A. Fagerlin, and P. A. Ubel. 2010. Risky feelings: Why a 6% risk of cancer doesn't always feel like 6%. *Patient Education and Counseling* 81(Suppl):S87-S93.

## ANNEX TO COMMISSIONED PAPER

### Estimating Quantitative Literacy Levels in U.S. Uninsured Adults

The percentage of Americans without health insurance in 2011 was 15.7 percent (U.S. Census Bureau, 2012). Using the 2003 National Assessment of Adult Literacy (NAAL) and 2009-2011 Census Bureau data, we calculated an estimate of the proportion of uninsured and insured American adults who fall into Below Basic, Basic, Intermediate, and Proficient quantitative literacy categories. The 2009-2011 Census Bureau provides data on the proportion of uninsured adults at each level of educational attainment (see Table Annex A-1), whereas the 2003 NAAL provides data on the proportion of adults in each quantitative literacy level by highest educational attainment (see Table Annex A-2). The NAAL sample consists of people ages 16 years and older living in households or prisons, whereas the sample of uninsured from the 2009-2011 Census consists of non-institutionalized civilian adults ages 25 and older. Thus, our comparison is imperfect, although it nonetheless gives an idea of the relative difference in quantitative literacy skills in patients and consumers that the health care system sees now (insured adults) and will likely see soon (previously uninsured adults). Additionally, according to the 2009-2011 Census, less than 1 percent (0.8 percent) of the uninsured population is age 65 and older; as a

**TABLE ANNEX A-1** 2009-2011 Census Bureau Data

| Civilian Non-Institutionalized Population 25 Years and Over | U.S. Population | Margin | Uninsured | Margin |
|---|---|---|---|---|
|  | 200,227,629 | ±23,788 | 31,883,520 | ±127,723 |
| Educational attainment |  |  |  |  |
| Less than high school graduate | 14.1% | ±0.1 | 27.2% | ±0.1 |
| High school graduate, GED, or alternative | 28.3% | ±0.1 | 34.1% | ±0.1 |
| Some college or associate's degree | 29.0% | ±0.1 | 26.9% | ±0.1 |
| Bachelor's degree or higher | 28.6% | ±0.1 | 11.9% | ±0.1 |
|  | 100.0% |  | 100.1% |  |

**TABLE ANNEX A-2** 2003 NAAL Quantitative Literacy Levels by Education

| Educational Attainment | Below Basic | Basic | Intermediate | Proficient | Total |
|---|---|---|---|---|---|
| Less than/some high school | 64.0% | 25.0% | 10.0% | 1.0% | 100.0% |
| High school graduate | 24.0% | 42.0% | 29.0% | 5.0% | 100.0% |
| Some college | 10.0% | 36.0% | 43.0% | 11.0% | 100.0% |
| Bachelor's degree | 4.0% | 22.0% | 43.0% | 31.0% | 100.0% |

result, our estimated proportions in the uninsured group would not change drastically if we had been able exclude older adults.

Among uninsured adults, we estimated that 28.8 percent are at the Below Basic level, 33.4 percent are at the Basic level, 29.3 percent are at the Intermediate level, and 8.6 percent are at the Proficient level (see Table Annex A-3). We calculated this estimate first by multiplying the proportion of uninsured adults at each level of education attainment (from Table Annex A-1) by the proportion of adults in each quantitative level at every level of education attainment (from Table Annex A-2). Next, we summed the proportions within each quantitative literacy level (across education levels) to get a total estimate of the proportion of uninsured at each level (see Table Annex A-3).

To estimate the proportion of insured adults who fall into each quantitative literacy category, we used the same procedure. We first calculated the proportion of insured adults at each level of education by using Table

**TABLE ANNEX A-3** Proportion of Uninsured Adults at Each Quantitative Literacy Level

| Educational Attainment | Below Basic | Basic | Intermediate | Proficient | Total |
|---|---|---|---|---|---|
| Less than/some high school | 17.4% | 6.8% | 2.7% | 0.3% | |
| High school graduate | 8.2% | 14.3% | 9.9% | 1.7% | |
| Some college | 2.7% | 9.7% | 11.6% | 3.0% | |
| Bachelor's degree | 0.5% | 2.6% | 5.1% | 3.7% | |
| % uninsured adults at each quantitative literacy level | 28.8% | 33.4% | 29.3% | 8.6% | 100.1% |

Annex A-1. We subtracted the number of uninsured adults from the U.S. population for each education level, and then divided that number by the total number of insured adults. Next, we followed the same multiplication and summation computations previously described with the uninsured population, but used the insured proportions.

# Appendix B

# Meeting Agenda

**Health Literacy and Numeracy: A Workshop**

**Keck 100**
**500 Fifth Street, NW**
**Washington, DC**

July 18, 2013          OPEN SESSION                    Room 100

8:30–8:40          Welcome and Introduction of First Two Speakers
                   *Paul Schyve, M.D.*
                   *Senior Advisor*
                   *The Joint Commission*

8:40–9:50          An Overview of Numeracy

8:40–9:00          What Is Numeracy?: It's More Than Mathematics
                   *Lynda Ginsburg, Ph.D.*
                   *Department of Mathematics*
                   *Rutgers University*

9:00–9:20          Presentation of Commissioned Paper. This
                   presentation will cover (1) what research shows about
                   people's numeracy skill levels; (2) what kinds of
                   numeracy skills are needed in health, e.g., selecting a
                   health plan, choosing treatments, and understanding
                   medication instructions; and (3) what we know about
                   how providers should communicate with those with
                   low numeracy skills.
                   *Ellen Peters, Ph.D.*
                   *Department of Psychology*
                   *Ohio State University*

| 9:20–9:50 | Discussion |
|---|---|
| 9:50–9:55 | Introduction of Speaker |

9:55–10:15      Are Numeracy Issues More Difficult with Poor
Health?
*Terry Davis, Ph.D.*
*Professor of Medicine and Pediatrics*
*Louisiana State University Health Sciences Center,*
*Shreveport*

| 10:15–10:30 | Discussion |
|---|---|
| 10:30–10:45 | BREAK |
| 10:45–10:55 | Introduction of Exercise and Panel Speakers |

10:55–11:00      Deconstruction Exercise
*Rima Rudd, Sc.D., M.S.P.H.*
*Department of Society, Human Development, and
Health*
*Harvard School of Public Health*

11:00–12:15      Numeracy Demands, Assumptions, and Challenges
for Consumers. These presentations will go into
more detail than background overview for each area
identified.

11:00–11:20      Choosing a Health Plan (will begin with a short video)
*Lynn Quincy, M.S.*
*Senior Policy Analyst*
*Consumers Union*

11:20–11:40      Numeracy in Health Care
*Andrea Apter, M.D., M.A., M.Sc.*
*Professor of Medicine*
*University of Pennsylvania*

| 11:40–12:15 | Discussion |
|---|---|
| 12:15–1:30 | MEMBER and SPEAKER LUNCH |

| 1:30–1:40 | Introduction of Panel |
|---|---|
| 1:40–3:00 | Panel: Numeracy Demands, Assumptions, and Challenges for Communicators. These presentations will go into more detail than background overview for each area identified. |
| 1:40–2:00 | Issues and Challenges Related to Journalism. This presentation will focus on how news organizations convey numerical information.<br>*Marguerite Holloway, M.S.*<br>*Assistant Professor*<br>*Columbia University Graduate School of Journalism* |
| 2:00–2:20 | Issues and Challenges in the Era of Shared Decision Making: Explaining Risk and Uncertainty<br>*Jessica S. Ancker, Ph.D., M.P.H.*<br>*Assistant Professor*<br>*Weill Cornell Medical College* |
| 2:20–3:00 | Discussion |
| 3:00–3:15 | BREAK |
| 3:15–3:25 | Introduction of Panel Presenters |
| 3:25–4:45 | Panel: Effective Strategies |
| 3:25–3:45 | Examples of Effective Display of Health Plan Information<br>*Robert M. Krughoff, J.D.*<br>*President, Center for the Study of Services*<br>*Consumers' CHECKBOOK* |
| 3:45–4:05 | Communicating Quantitative Information for Decision Making<br>*Brian Zikmund-Fisher, Ph.D.*<br>*Assistant Professor, School of Public Health*<br>*University of Michigan* |

| 4:05–4:25 | Effectively Communicating Medication Instructions |
|-----------|---------------------------------------------------|
|           | *Michael Wolf, Ph.D., M.P.H.* |
|           | *Associate Professor* |
|           | *Northwestern University Feinberg School of Medicine* |

4:25–4:45    Discussion

4:45–4:55    Exercise Results

4:55–5:30    Reflections on the Day

5:30         ADJOURN

# Appendix C

# Speaker Biosketches

**Jessica S. Ancker, Ph.D., M.P.H.,** is an assistant professor in the Center for Healthcare Informatics and Policy at Weill Cornell Medical College in New York City. She uses quantitative and qualitative methods to study how health information technology (HIT) affects decisions, behaviors, and outcomes. Her research interests lie at the intersection of human factors research, decision science, and health literacy. Recent publications and ongoing projects focus on health numeracy, risk communication, data visualization for patients as well as physicians, and decision support. She is the recipient of an Agency for Healthcare Research and Quality (AHRQ) K award to examine ways in which electronic patient portals can be better adapted to support comprehension and decision making. In addition, Dr. Ancker conducts a complementary set of research activities involving the evaluation of the effects of HIT. She is a deputy director of HITEC (the Health Information Technology Evaluation Collaborative), a multi-institutional research collaborative directed by Dr. Rainu Kaushal at Weill Cornell. Her HITEC projects have included surveys of technology adoption and attitudes, usability evaluation, and mixed-method approaches to studying the effects of the nation's unprecedented movement toward electronic health records.

Her current position reflects a career that has focused on effective communication of complex information in a variety of ways. Her first career was in journalism and writing, including positions as an Associated Press reporter and as the manager of medical editing at the Cleveland Clinic. As a writer, she became fascinated with the ways in which quantitative information was used and misused in decision making. After earning her M.P.H.

from the Department of Biostatistics at Columbia University, she completed her Ph.D. from the Department of Biomedical Informatics with the support of a National Library of Medicine (NLM) Fellowship. She worked with a multidisciplinary dissertation committee composed of a behavioral scientist, a decision scientist, and an informaticist/linguist. Dr. Ancker is also a dedicated educator, with experience teaching biostatistics, scientific writing, statistical graphics, and informatics. The program director for the Weill Cornell Health Information Technology Certificate, Dr. Ancker was awarded the Excellence in Teaching Award at Weill Cornell in 2013. She continues to guest lecture on statistical literacy issues for journalists.

**Andrea Apter, M.D., M.A., M.Sc.,** received her bachelor's degree with high honors from the University of Connecticut, where she was a University Scholar and a member of Phi Beta Kappa. She then earned a master's degree in mathematics from Temple University and taught mathematics in secondary school before entering medical school. After receiving an M.D. from the University of Pennsylvania, she completed a residency in Internal Medicine and a Fellowship in Allergy and Immunology at Northwestern University School of Medicine. She practiced general medicine in a rural community for 1 year and then joined the faculty of the University of Connecticut Health Center. There she developed an interest in clinical research related to asthma that led to completion of an M.S. in epidemiology from the Harvard School of Public Health. In 1998 she moved to the University of Pennsylvania. Dr. Apter's research focuses on asthma, the environmental and social factors that influence disease, patient–clinician communication including electronic communication, and the impact of health literacy on health, all with the goal of reducing health disparities. She has been the recipient of funding for research from the National Heart, Lung, and Blood Institute, which has included research grants and two career development awards, one focused on health literacy's contribution to health. Dr. Apter's interest in health literacy evolved from her experiences as a school teacher, and then working with patients and the realization that limited educational opportunities affect the acquisition of health care and the self-management of chronic diseases, including asthma. With her collaborators she validated a measure of numeracy specific for asthma patients, the Asthma Numeracy Questionnaire. She has used it to explore the relationship of numeracy and health and to develop interventions to allow patients to overcome barriers to literacy that might affect access to care and patient–physician communication. Current projects examine electronic literacy and health communication.

Dr. Apter is an associate editor of the *Journal of Allergy and Clinical Immunology*; she served on the Food and Drug Administration (FDA) Pulmonary Allergy Drug Advisory Committee and as a director of the American Board of Allergy and Immunology. She is currently a board member of the American Academy of Allergy, Asthma and Immunology (AAAAI). She has been named a *U.S. News & World Report*'s Top Doctor, Top Doc by *Philadelphia* magazine, and Distinguished Clinician by the AAAAI.

**Terry C. Davis, Ph.D.,** a pioneer in the field of health literacy, is a professor of medicine and pediatrics at Louisiana State University Health Sciences Center in Shreveport. For the past 25 years, she has been studying the impact of patient literacy on health and health care. Seminal achievements include development of the Rapid Estimate of Adult Literacy in Medicine (REALM) and creation of user-friendly patient education and provider training materials that are being used nationally. Dr. Davis has more than 120 publications related to health literacy and health communication. She has served on Health Literacy Advisory Boards for both the American Medical Association (AMA) and the American College of Physicians (ACP). She was an independent agent on the Institute of Medicine (IOM) Committee on Health Literacy and a developer of the AMA's Train-the-Trainer Health Literacy Curriculum. Currently she is a member of the Healthy People 2020 Health Literacy/Health Communication Section and serves as a health literacy advisor to the FDA.

Dr. Davis is the Health Literacy Principal Investigator (PI) on a National Institutes of Health grant for the Louisiana Clinical and Translational Science Center, an unprecedented collaborative effort among eight academic institutions in Louisiana. She is PI on a 5-year National Cancer Institute (NCI) health literacy intervention to increase regular breast and colorectal cancer screening among patients in Federally Qualified Health Centers. Building on this work, she was recently awarded an American Cancer Society (ACS) grant to evaluate follow-up strategies to improve regular colorectal cancer screening in rural clinics in the state. Dr. Davis is also working with Drs. Mike Wolf and Ruth Parker on AHRQ-funded studies to improve patient understanding and actual use of prescription medication labels in English and Spanish. Along with a team from the University of North Carolina and University of California, San Francisco, she has been funded by the ACP to develop and test practical self-management guides and videos for patients with diabetes, chronic obstructive pulmonary disease, coronary artery disease, obesity, and rheumatoid arthritis. The ACP has distributed more than 5 million copies of these guides.

**Lynda Ginsburg, Ph.D.,** is a senior research associate for mathematics education and associate director at the Center for Mathematics, Science and Computer Education at Rutgers University. Her research interests include mathematics education for adult populations, intergenerational mathematics learning, and adult teacher professional learning. She is currently the associate director of a Math–Science Partnership project funded by the National Science Foundation (NSF), New Jersey Partnership for Excellence in Middle School Mathematics. For the recently completed Department of Education/OVAE Adult Numeracy Instruction project, she was lead author of the *Guidelines for Adult Numeracy Instruction* and evaluated the project's professional development initiative. She conducted research on parent involvement in mathematics learning in urban settings for the recently completed, NSF-funded CLT, *MetroMath: The Center for Mathematics in America's Cities*. Previously, she was a senior researcher at the National Center on Adult Literacy at the University of Pennsylvania for 12 years, directing or contributing to a number of national research and professional development projects. She has served on numerous national advisory groups, was a founding member of the Adult Numeracy Network, designs and provides professional development on numeracy for multiple states, and has published and presented her work nationally and internationally. Dr. Ginsburg holds a Ph.D. in urban education/mathematics education from the University of Wisconsin–Milwaukee and has taught mathematics or mathematics education at the high school, adult education, and university levels.

**Marguerite Holloway, M.S.,** is the director of science and environmental journalism and a professor at Columbia University's Graduate School of Journalism, where she has been teaching since 1997. For many years, Holloway codirected a dual-degree program in Earth and Environmental Science Journalism; in 2004, she designed the science and health reporting curriculum for the M.A. program, a new degree that was launched in 2005-2006 to provide subject-area expertise to experienced journalists. That M.A. course today, known as the Robert Wood Johnson Foundation Program in Health and Science Journalism, is cotaught by experts in various fields. Holloway was a long-time editor and writer at *Scientific American*, where she covered public health, women in science, neuroscience, and natural history, and where she worked closely with researchers on their articles. She has written for many other publications as well, including *The New York Times*, the *Village Voice*, and *Discover*, and began her career as a reporter for a medical biweekly. Her first book, *The Measure of Manhattan*, which tells the story of the exacting, irascible, and colorful surveyor and inventor who laid the grid on New York City, was published earlier this year by W.W. Norton. Holloway has a B.S. from Brown University and an M.S. from Columbia.

**Robert Krughoff, J.D.,** is president of the Center for the Study of Services/ Consumers' CHECKBOOK, an independent, nonprofit consumer information organization whose mission since 1974 has been to educate and inform consumers to help them select and deal with service providers, including individual health care providers (doctors, hospitals, dentists, etc.) and insurers (auto, homeowners, health). For more than 33 years, the organization has published *Guide to Health Plans for Federal Employees and Retirees*, a health plan comparison tool. The organization's publications and websites have been supported by individual consumers who find the information useful enough that they pay for access. Krughoff has been responsible for developing measures of service quality and cost and assessing which are of greatest interest and usability for consumers (e.g., which measures of physician quality and health plan cost and quality), and has documented widespread market failures.

Krughoff has served on the board of directors of the Consumer Federation of America, the board of directors of Consumers Union/*Consumer Reports*, and advisory and study panels for the Institute of Medicine, Agency for Healthcare Research and Quality, National Quality Forum, and other organizations. He has been the recipient of the National Press Club's First Place Award for Excellence in Consumer Journalism, the Esther Peterson Consumer Service Award from the Consumer Federation of America, the Consumer Advocate award from the National Association of Consumer Agency Administrators, and the annual Friend of Consumer Award from the American Council on Consumer Interests. A graduate of Amherst College and University of Chicago Law School, Krughoff early in his career served as special assistant to the Assistant Secretary for Planning and Evaluation and then as director of the Office of Research and Evaluation Planning at the U.S. Department of Health and Human Services (HHS; then the U.S. Department of Health, Education, and Welfare).

**Ellen Peters, Ph.D.,** is a professor in Ohio State University's (OSU's) Department of Psychology. She graduated from the University of Pennsylvania with bachelor's degrees in engineering and marketing and earned her Ph.D. in psychology from the University of Oregon. She joined Decision Research in 1998 and was promoted to senior research scientist in 2006. In 2010, she became an associate professor in OSU's Psychology Department and was promoted to professor in 2012. Dr. Peters is a recognized leader in risk perception/communication and the psychology of health decision making, publishing papers on the effects of affect, numeracy, number processing, and aging. With more than 80 peer-reviewed publications, her research focuses on how affective, intuitive, and deliberative processes help people to make decisions in an increasingly complex world. She is a Fellow of the American Psychological Society and has worked extensively with federal agencies (e.g., NCI, FDA) to advance the science of human decision making as it applies to health decisions and communication. In particular, she was a founding member of the FDA's Risk Communication Advisory

Committee and has chaired that committee. She has also been a consultant to the FDA's Tobacco Products Scientific Advisory Committee, and she has worked extensively with the design of decision aids to maximize their comprehension and use across diverse populations.

**Lynn Quincy, M.S.,** is a senior health policy analyst for Consumers Union, the policy and advocacy division of *Consumer Reports*. Ms. Quincy works on a wide variety of health policy issues, with a particular focus on consumer protections, consumers' health insurance literacy, and health insurance reform at the federal and state levels. Her recent work includes studies testing consumer reactions to new health insurance disclosure forms; launching an initiative to measure consumers' health insurance literacy; a study that explores approaches to actuarial value estimation; and a study that examines the use of "choice architecture" in health plan chooser tools. Work in progress includes consumer testing explanations of the new health premium tax credit. Ms. Quincy also serves as a consumer expert in several venues: as a consumer representative with the National Association of Insurance Commissioners, a member of the Covered California Plan Management Advisory Workgroup, and on the technical expert panel advising the development of new exchange enrollee satisfaction surveys.

Prior to joining Consumers Union, Ms. Quincy held senior positions with Mathematica Policy Research, Inc., the Institute for Health Policy Solutions, and Watson Wyatt Worldwide (now Towers Watson). She holds a master's degree in economics from the University of Maryland.

**Rima Rudd, Sc.D., M.S.P.H.,** is the senior lecturer on health literacy, education, and policy at the Harvard School of Public Health. Her work centers on health communication and on the design and evaluation of public health community-based programs. She has been teaching courses on innovative strategies in health education, program planning and evaluation, psychosocial and behavioral theory, and health literacy since 1988. Dr. Rudd is focusing her research inquiries and policy work on literacy related–disparities and literacy-related barriers to health programs, services, and care, working closely with the adult education, public health, oral health, and medical sectors.

Dr. Rudd wrote several reports that helped shape the agenda in health literacy research and practice. They include the health literacy chapter of the HHS report *Communicating Health: Priorities and Strategies for Progress* (2003) and the 2010 *National Call for Action*. She coded all health-related items in the international surveys for assessments of adult literacy skills enabling Australia, Canada, New Zealand, and the United States and other countries to assess national health literacy skills. She authored the Educational Testing Services report *Literacy and Health in America* (2004) and contributed to other national assessments. Dr. Rudd provided two in-depth literature reviews (*Review of Adult Learning and Literacy* volume 1 in 2000 and volume 7 in 2007). She served on the IOM Committee on Health Literacy, the National Research Council Committee on Measuring Adult Literacy, the National Institute of Dental and Craniofacial Research Workgroup on Oral Health Literacy, and the Joint Commission Advisory Committee on Health Literacy and Patient Safety. She also contributed to the ensuing reports and white papers as well as to several IOM Roundtable on Health Literacy publications. She has received national and international awards for her work in health literacy. Most recently, the University of Maryland named a doctoral scholar's award in her honor.

**Michael S. Wolf, M.A., M.P.H., Ph.D.,** is professor of medicine, associate division chief (Internal Medicine and Geriatrics), and director of the Health Literacy & Learning Program (HeLP) within the Feinberg School of Medicine, Northwestern University. He also holds appointments in Cognitive Sciences, Communication Studies, Medical Social Science, Psychiatry, and Surgery. As a behavioral scientist and health services researcher, Dr. Wolf has extensively studied cognitive and psychosocial determinants of health, specifically in the area of health literacy and health communications research. His work has focused primarily on deconstructing self-care tasks and understanding health care complexity. Dr. Wolf has led several large-scale, real-world controlled trials to evaluate multifaceted interventions to promote patient engagement in health, targeting use of clinical preventive services, chronic disease self-management, and medication safety and adherence. He is the PI of the National Institute on Aging–funded cohort study referred to as LitCog, which examines the associations among reading, numeracy, and an expanse of cognitive abilities and their influence on health behavior.

**Brian Zikmund-Fisher, Ph.D.,** is an assistant professor in the Department of Health Behavior and Health Education, University of Michigan (UM) School of Public Health and a research assistant professor in the UM Department of Internal Medicine. In addition, he is affiliated with the UM Center for Bioethics and Social Sciences in Medicine, the UM Risk Science Center, and the UM Health Informatics Program.

Dr. Zikmund-Fisher received his Ph.D. in behavioral decision theory (a combination of decision psychology and behavioral economics) from Carnegie Mellon University. He uses this interdisciplinary background to study factors that affect individuals' ability to use data to inform their health and medical decision making. An author of more than 75 articles and book chapters, Dr. Zikmund-Fisher researches the design of formats and visual displays to make health risk and test data more intuitively meaningful and studies the effects of numeracy (people's ability to use numbers to inform their health decisions) on health communication. His projects have included the National Survey of Medical Decisions (often called the DECISIONS Study), a grant funded by the National Institute of Environmental Health Sciences, studying perceptions of risk from dioxin exposure within affected communities; an ACS award regarding the development and testing of visual displays of risk; and several small projects examining how patient testimonials influence risk perceptions and decision making. At UM, Dr. Zikmund-Fisher teaches graduate courses in risk communication and designing health messages.